1 POUND
A DAY

1 POUND
A DAY

❦

THE MARTHA'S VINEYARD DIET DETOX AND PLAN FOR A LIFETIME OF HEALTHY EATING

Dr. Roni DeLuz, RN, ND, PhD,
and James Hester

with Diane Reverand

G

GALLERY BOOKS

New York London Toronto Sydney New Delhi

G

Gallery Books
A Division of Simon & Schuster, Inc.
1230 Avenue of the Americas
New York, NY 10020

First Gallery Books paperback edition March 2014

GALLERY BOOKS and colophon
are registered trademarks of Simon & Schuster, Inc.

For information about special discounts for bulk purchases,
please contact Simon & Schuster Special Sales
at 1-866-506-1949 or business@simonandschuster.com.

The Simon & Schuster Speakers Bureau can bring authors
to your live event. For more information or to book
an event contact the Simon & Schuster Speakers Bureau
at 1-866-248-3049 or visit our website at www.simonspeakers.com.

Designed by Julie Schroeder

Manufactured in the United States of America

1   3   5   7   9   10   8   6   4   2

The Library of Congress has cataloged the hardcover edition as follows:

DeLuz, Roni.
1 pound a day : the Martha's Vineyard diet detox and plan for a lifetime of
healthy eating / by Dr. Roni DeLuz, R.N., N.D., Ph.D., and James Hester ;
with Diane Reverand. — First Gallery Books hardcover edition.
pages   cm
1. Detoxification (Health)   2. Reducing diets—Recipes.   I. Hester,
James.   II. Reverand, Diane.   III. Title.   IV. Title: One pound a day.
RA784.5.D45 2013
613.2'5—dc23   2013000497

ISBN 978-1-4767-2744-8
ISBN 978-1-4767-2745-5 (pbk)
ISBN 978-1-4767-2746-2 (ebook)

We dedicate this book with love and appreciation to all our detox graduates. Your stories, questions, challenges, and successes have inspired us to write our second book. You have made this book possible because your histories helped to lay the foundation.

MEDICAL DISCLAIMER

Roni DeLuz is not a medical physician, psychologist, or pharmacist. Neither is James Hester. Roni DeLuz is a registered nurse, a PhD in natural health, a lifestyle consultant, and a certified colon hydrotherapist.

This publication contains the opinions and ideas of its authors. It is a source of information only and is sold with the understanding that the authors and publisher are not engaged in rendering medical, health, or any other kind of personal professional services in the book. The reader should consult his or her medical, health, or other competent professional before adopting any of the suggestions in this book; beginning any diet detox, detox, or diet plan; or taking any herbs or supplements.

The authors and publisher specifically disclaim all responsibility for any liability, loss, or risk, personal or otherwise, which is incurred as a consequence, directly or indirectly, of the use and application of any of the ideas and information in this book.

Give Us Thirty Days,
and We'll Change Your Life

1 Pound a Day will change your life. That is not an empty promise. It is what we hear from everyone who does the program. Whether they come to the retreat on Martha's Vineyard or do the detox on their own with the help of our first book, the *New York Times* bestseller *21 Pounds in 21 Days*, thousands of people have had fantastic results. They call, write to us, post testimonials on Facebook and our website, and tweet about just how great they feel. They cannot stop talking about how the detox has transformed them. They go from being exhausted, overweight, down, and sick to seeing a huge improvement in just thirty days. They lighten up in every way. They lose a pound a day, their energy soars, and their spirits are higher than ever. We'll share their success stories throughout *1 Pound a Day*, along with their tips on what they do to make detoxing easy and—yes—even fun. Their insights on the process will smooth the way for you. You will see how thrilled 1 Pound a Day detoxers are by the changes in their looks and health. They are proud of what they have accomplished. They deserve to be.

Our new book, *1 Pound a Day*, offers an expanded, simplified month-long program to rid your body of toxins, and a new plan for keeping it clean for the rest of your life. Since our first book was published six years ago, we have spent a lot of our time giving support to people all over the world undergoing the detox at home. Judging from the hundreds of questions we receive each month, we have learned exactly where detoxers need direction. We have come to see that if you are detoxing at home, not only do you need a program that is simpler than what we offer at the retreat, where there is a staff of professionals to support you, but you need more guidelines, tips, and recipes.

Doing this detox should not become a part-time job. We have streamlined the detox and made it more practical. We provide tips and suggestions from our own experience as well as from other detoxers to guarantee a month of detoxing that will run like clockwork. You will learn to make fresh juices and soups that appeal to you from recipes created for various palates. We tell you how to order online the supplements we use at the retreat, as we did in our first book, and suggest products that are readily available at your local vitamin or health food store.

> This is a lifestyle . . . What you get out of this detox that you don't get from other diets is your health. It is the rebuilding of your body. I am talking about the whole, total rejuvenation. Nothing else promises or offers that.
>
> Robin Quivers

Based on what we have learned from people who have done the program, it has become clear to us that detoxers need more help transitioning from the detox back to normal eating. That is why we have changed the program from twenty-one days to thirty. The transition back to normal eating is a very important part of permanent weight loss and continued health improvements. Doing a detox is not like flipping an on-off switch—on the detox and then back to junk food. You do not want to shock your digestive system by going out and bingeing on chips, pizza, and chocolate on day twenty-two. Reintroducing food to your cleansed system should be a gradual process. We will walk you through that nine-day period, giving you a specific plan to help you ease back into a less restricted diet. This part of the program will lock in the changes you have experienced and set you on the right path for sustained good health.

Yo-yo dieting is proof of how hard it is to keep weight off and make healthy eating a habit. Once you have made up your mind, it is not so difficult to follow a specific set of food rules for a month. It just takes a little discipline. You do not have many choices. That is the retreat mentality. When you are on your own after thirty days, the temptations can be a lot more challenging. Your commitment to health does not end in a month. If you want to continue to look and feel terrific, you have to eat clean. In this book, we want to pay more attention to where the real change has to happen—how you eat after you are done detoxing.

We give you guidelines and strategies for eating in the most nutritious way possible every day, so that your post-detox glow and restored energy are permanent. Dr. Roni has five basic principles for wholesome eating that will make eating right a habit. We have supplied two weeks of daily eating plans that offer a variety of breakfasts, lunches, snacks, dinners, and desserts that are so satisfying that your food cravings will vanish. We include delicious, healthy recipes from Dr. Roni's kitchen. These dishes are sophisticated and represent a broad range of cuisines and eating styles. The recipes will convince you that eating healthy does not have to be bland or boring.

We are realists. No one is perfect. There are times when we all backslide. Dr. Roni's 75/25 formula gives you room to have that piece of fried chicken or dish of ice cream every now and then. If you can eat well 75 percent of the time, you are doing great. If you really go off the rails, we provide two-day and seven-day detoxes to get you back in control of your eating.

The three parts of this book are designed to help you return to health and to stay at peak levels of well-being. Our program is so much more than a diet, as you will see in the pages that follow. Part 1, Want to Get Light?, will motivate you to clean up your act. Starting with the scary facts, we will explain what toxins and bad food choices are doing to your body. Then we will show you how detoxing restores your health. Along the way, we quote from people who told us about their experiences on our Facebook pages or in other communications to us.

The second part, The 1 Pound a Day Diet Detox, is a step-by-step guide to the new and revised diet detox. It starts with a daily plan for the first twenty-one days of the detox. We explain the benefits of the supplements, juices, broths, and soups that constitute the program. We introduce techniques that will speed up and deepen the detoxification process. Two chapters contain recipes for highly nutritious juices, broths, and soups. Part 2 will end with the final, all-important stage of the detox: a nine-day transition plan to take you gently back to everyday eating.

Keep It Going, the last part of the book, will give you a blueprint for eating clean every day of your life—to nourish your body on a cellular level and to maintain super energy and excellent health. Dr. Roni explains what it means to eat clean and outlines her health maintenance diet. We cover the crucial importance of keeping your body in balance and advise you on how to avoid an acidic biochemistry. We even show you how to turn up your metabolism. For those times when you lose your resolve, we detail abbreviated versions of the detox to get you back on track. The book will end with meal plans and delicious, healthy recipes that will inspire you to change the way you eat for life. Although the pounds will evaporate, the benefits of the 1 Pound a Day Diet Detox go way beyond weight loss. We want to move into the territory of long-term change and healing.

We know what the detox can do because it has changed—or more accurately saved—our own lives. Dr. Roni developed the detox to heal herself. She had a Bachelor of Science in Nursing from Fairfield University. She owned and operated three nursing homes in Southern California that provided health care to medically fragile and developmentally disabled children. In 1989, she became so sick she could barely get out of bed. Her health had been on a downward spiral over a period of two years. What started as feeling a bit off evolved into having increasingly frequent headaches and feeling pain in her joints. Though she lived on aspirin or Tylenol to relieve the pain, her symptoms intensified. As she went from one specialist to another, her list of prescription drugs grew longer. She was taking seven different drugs but just kept getting worse. Whatever was wrong with her was taking over her body and her life, and none of the specialists could come up with an explanation. They just kept prescribing more medications. What happened next is best described by Dr. Roni:

I thought I was going to die. Since traditional medicine was not helping, I turned to alternative treatments. I went to see an herbalist who treated illness with plant-based remedies. When I described my symptoms, he explained that my body was being compromised by a toxic overload. I learned I had been poisoning myself with all the medications prescribed by the nearly thirty specialists I had seen. My digestive system was in bad shape. The herbalist recommended that I eat organic baby food, which was easier to digest and far more nutritious than the diet I had been eating. In three months, my energy was returning, and I felt stronger. As the doctor gradually weaned me off the prescription drugs, I improved even more.

At the recommendation of the doctor who had helped me so much, I went to American Biologics in Tijuana, Mexico, for virus tests, which revealed that my liver was compromised. I was diagnosed with chronic fatigue syndrome (CFS) and fibromyalgia. In retrospect, I realize I had been suffering from environmental illness.

Once I returned to California, I learned everything I could about holistic medicine. I began to understand how the body heals itself naturally. I learned to teach the chronically ill how to create the right conditions in the body for natural healing. I earned my naturopathic doctor (ND) Certification and a PhD in natural health from Clayton College and the Holistic College of Nutrition.

I developed the cleansing program and healing philosophy behind *1 Pound a Day* while nursing myself back to top health.

In 1999, I moved back east and opened the Martha's Vineyard Holistic Retreat, where I taught my clients how to repair, regenerate, and rejuvenate themselves by detoxifying their bodies. To the delight of my clients, we discovered that weight loss was a side effect of the detoxification process.

In 2003, James Hester came to the retreat to lose weight. He had hit a bad patch in his life personally and professionally and had put on more than forty pounds. I guided him through my program twice, and he lost forty-three pounds. He was surprised that he looked so much younger. He replaced his anger with vibrancy. His energy level and attitude had returned to their optimal state.

He became a convert and wanted to get the message out. We collaborated to write a book. It went on to become the *New York Times* bestseller *21 Pounds in 21 Days* with the support of Wendy Williams, Robin Quivers, and Steve Harvey and James's appearances on *Larry King Live*, *The View*, and *CBS Sunday Morning*. James's passion got the word out, and the amazing results people got from the detox did the rest.

He has become my business partner and an expert on the practical aspects of the detox. James loves to detox and looks forward to the clean and clear feelings he experiences each time. He finds that doing a full detox three times a year works for him, with quick tune-ups when necessary. In the past ten years, he has done more than thirty detoxes himself and has guided hundreds of people through the process. He knows what it takes to stay on track and has a good time doing it. His experience will help to guide you through the process.

Since our book was published, we have watched juicing, cleanses, fasts, and detox diets become a part of popular culture. We were way ahead of the times. We know that this new health consciousness, this interest in ridding the body of toxins and eating clean, is more than a fad. Obesity has become the number one health concern in this country. The diseases that are killing us are linked to excess weight and the toxic load that throw our bodies out of balance and stress our organs. We know that when you commit to thirty days on the 1 Pound a Day Diet Detox, you will benefit immeasurably from the purest, freshest food and the deepest cleanse available. You owe yourself this chance to transform yourself and to look and feel great for the rest of your life.

Dr. Roni DeLuz and James Hester

CONTENTS

1 POUND
A DAY

NO CHEWING?
IT'S EASIER THAN YOU THINK

Just the thought of a detox probably sounds like deprivation to you. Doing the 1 Pound a Day Diet Detox does take commitment, but the payoff is worth the effort. Unless you try it, you will never know how great you can feel and how fabulous you will look when you flush out all the toxins that are stressing your body. Consider it a one-month adventure in uncharted territory that leads to the fountain of youth. Time and again we hear from our detoxers that the cleansing month flies by. It is an exciting time. The changes they experience so quickly create momentum and motivation to keep going.

You take time off or go on vacation to relax and restore yourself. It's a start, but don't you think your entire body deserves a major holiday, too? Give it a rest. That means more than just reducing everyday stress and getting enough sleep. You have to go deep to give your organs a break.

Mother Nature did not design your body to mop up the thousands of manmade chemicals that are poisoning you from the air you breathe, the water you drink, the food you eat, the cleaning and personal grooming products you use, even the clothes you wear. Toxic chemicals accumulate in your organs and make your body sluggish. Toxins affect the way your body metabolizes food and eliminates waste. The end result: those unwanted pounds. Unless you do something about it, toxic overload will overwhelm your body as it struggles to expel damaging chemicals, and you will eventually get sick.

Everything goes more smoothly when your house is in order. Commit yourself to discovering how light you can feel when you clean up from the inside out. You know how great it is to organize your closet and wardrobe and get rid of clothes you never wear that crowd your drawers and closets. Putting yourself together in the morning becomes a pleasure instead of a mad dash with clothing, accessories, and shoes tossed everywhere. The same is true for your body. It functions more smoothly when toxins do not jam up the works. We are offering you a way to take care of your body like the prized possession it is.

You will be amazed as your weight drops steadily. You will like what you see in the mirror— glowing skin, clear bright eyes, glossier hair. The 1 Pound a Day Diet Detox is the ultimate natural beauty treatment, but it has many other powerful benefits that will improve your life. People who have done the program have reported

> This detox has changed my life in every aspect! I completed the detox, and I lost 20.2 pounds! I have never in my life felt this great about my body and my overall health. I feel amazing!!!! I have lost inches all over my body and that has never happened to me with any other weight-loss program. My skin is so clean and clear, everyone tells me that I am glowing! All my clothes are falling off me. I have definitely added additional waking hours to my day. I am so full of energy that I no longer need naps. I haven't had any headaches, nausea (which was daily for me), gas, or heartburn.
>
> Jannica S. Covington

- Supercharged energy and less need to sleep or nap
- Better mental clarity, memory, focus
- Fewer headaches and backaches
- Reduction of arthritis, knee, and joint pain
- Fewer colds and a stronger immune system

- Reduction of cellulite
- Improved acne, eczema, and other skin conditions
- Breaking addictions for sugar, caffeine, and nicotine
- Slowing down hair loss
- Stronger fingernails and shining hair
- Reduction of digestive problems
- Restoration of regularity

1 Pound a Day will give you the tools you need to transform your life, to go from blah to radiant. Think of this cleansing detox as a jump start for lifestyle changes that will last forever.

TOXIC OVERLOAD TEST

Take this test to gauge your need to detox. We are exposed to so many toxins in our lives. Some things are beyond our control, but we have the capacity to change some of our lifestyle choices. This test will give you a sense of the toxic burden your body carries.

1. Where do you live?
    a. City
    b. Suburb
    c. Country

2. How is your weight? Are you:
    a. Obese
    b. Overweight
    c. Average to lean

3. Do you have a hard time losing weight and keeping it off?
    a. Yes
    b. Sometimes
    c. Never

4. How much processed food do you eat a day?
    a. 5 to 9 servings
    b. 2 to 4 servings
    c. 1 serving or less

5. How much water do you drink each day?
   a. 3 glasses or less
   b. 4 to 7 glasses
   c. 8 glasses or more

6. What is your level of stress?
   a. Extreme
   b. Moderate with some spikes
   c. Usually minimal

7. Do you use commercial household cleaners and personal grooming products?
   a. Use conventional products
   b. Use a mix of conventional and chemical-free
   c. Use organic and nontoxic products

8. Do you lose energy or get tired during the day?
   a. Often
   b. Sometimes
   c. Never

9. Is your mental state:
   a. Cloudy and fuzzy more than 50 percent of the time
   b. Mostly clear with occasional fog
   c. Sharp and crystal clear

10. Do you suffer from indigestion, stomach problems, frequent gas, bad breath, or irregularity?
    a. Frequently
    b. Sometimes
    c. Never

11. Do you experience food intolerances that give you postnasal drip, blurred vision, burping, headaches, itching, burning eyes, sneezing, swollen eyes, or a swollen face?
    a. Yes, from specific foods
    b. Sometimes
    c. Never

12. Do you experience insomnia?
    a. Yes
    b. Sometimes
    c. Never

If *a* is your answer to six or more of these questions, you urgently need to detox. Your current situation and your choices are increasing your toxic load and are already affecting your health and well-being. If you select *b* most often, toxins are probably draining you of energy and causing you discomfort. You should detox to keep poisonous chemicals from accumulating in your body and intensifying the physical symptoms and problems you might have. If you have a mix of *a* and *b* choices with very few *c*'s, your need to detox is more urgent. If your response to eight or more of these questions is *c*, you are on the right track to health. You could benefit from the 1 Pound a Day Diet Detox to increase your vitality and longevity.

The 1 Pound A Day Diet Detox not only cleanses the organs of your body of accumulated toxins but also nourishes your body on a cellular level. The terms "cleanse" and "detox" have become interchangeable, but there is a distinction. A cleanse primarily focuses on clearing the digestive tract, so that waste does not build up. Our detox eliminates toxins from the organs, the bloodstream, and the entire body, and replenishes the nutrients the body needs to heal and regenerate. This powerful detox uses fresh vegetable juices, pureed vegetable soups, homemade broths, teas, dried and liquid phytonutrients from green vegetables, and antioxidants to fight inflammation, improve joint health, and boost the immune system; probiotics to enhance digestion; and antiaging compounds. Get ready not to chew for twenty-one days, and then to add solid food in a very controlled way during the next nine. Not eating solid food for that length of time might seem challenging, but your or-

> My exclusive focus on weight loss as a by-product of the detox changed dramatically after visiting my MD for an annual checkup. My labs were all normal, and I'm off cholesterol medication for over one year. My heart is efficient, more so than ever before. I have not had a bout with seasonal allergies in more than a year.
>
> Patti Firrincili

gans need a rest. Your body needs to repair itself from toxic damage while getting maximum nutrition. Thirty minutes a day of gentle exercise will support the detox process. We are not suggesting that you do a hard workout at the gym or go to a fast-paced aerobics class. That would stress your body too much while you are detoxing. Instead, we recommend a thirty-minute walk or yoga session each day. You can break your exercise into two fifteen-minute walks or sessions if that works better for you.

In the purifying process of the detox, normal hunger disappears as your organs do the work of cleansing. When you provide your body with the nutrients it needs on a cellular level, you will be surprised to see that your appetite changes. Hunger pangs and unhealthy food cravings vanish.

If you are not yet persuaded that detoxing is for you, the first chapter, Why Detox?, will convince you how important a deep cleanse is for your health. If detoxing seems like something wacko that health fanatics do, that chapter will change your mind. By the time you finish reading it, you will be determined to flush toxins from your system, lose weight, and transform your life.

PART 1

~

WANT TO GET LIGHT?

CHAPTER 1

WHY DETOX?

You are exposed to toxins and noxious substances everywhere you turn. More than 80,000 man-made chemicals have been introduced since World War II, and most of those have never been tested for safety. Your body does not experience these toxins one at a time. No one knows the effects of the potentially harmful interactions of these chemicals that you encounter every second. No matter how hard you try, you cannot avoid toxic exposure. Toxins are so much more pervasive than you think. When you consider pollution, the earth's atmosphere, soil, and water automatically come to mind. You accept that industrial waste and car emissions do a lot of damage, but you may not be aware that you live in a toxic stew in your own home. The fact is that the inside of your house is more toxic than outside. Almost all modern conveniences and items you use without a second thought contain harmful chemicals. What follows is a list of some of the products with highly toxic ingredients or components.

Synthetic fabrics are petroleum based and processed with many chemicals.

Residues from pesticides are found in conventionally grown vegetables and fruit.

Conventionally raised meat and poultry contain pesticides from feed, plus antibiotics and hormones.

Fish are contaminated with dangerous levels of mercury.

Processed food is loaded with additives, preservatives, and coloring.

Carpets and upholstered furniture outgas formaldehyde and other toxins.

Vinyl flooring is toxic.

Mattresses contain flame retardants by law; those chemicals are neurotoxins.

Wrinkle-resistant, stain-resistant, drip-dry fabrics all have toxic finishes.

Paint contains highly toxic solvents and volatile organic compounds.

Polyurethane finishes outgas toxic fumes.

Home cleaning products contain a host of toxic ingredients.

Grooming products and cosmetics are filled with chemicals that are absorbed through your skin or inhaled in a mist.

Nonstick pots and pans can be deadly.

Pressed or treated wood used to make furniture and cabinets outgases formaldehyde.

Dry cleaning fluid residues are powerful neurotoxins.

Food cans are lined with plastic that leaches chemicals into the contents.

Plastic food containers, food packaging, and wraps contain highly toxic phthalates and BPA.

Plastic toys can be toxic unless labeled "BPA-free."

Cell phones, computers, televisions, and microwaves disrupt electromagnetic fields and outgas BPAs and other harmful chemicals.

These items and countless more are part of your everyday life. Toxins enter your body from the air you breathe, the water you drink, and what you eat, and are absorbed through your skin. Your body is not designed to process this avalanche of man-made chemicals.

Relentless exposure to synthetic chemicals increases your toxic load to levels your body is not equipped to handle. The accumulation of toxins overwhelms your body, disrupting normal functions. Toxins are silent killers, and diseases are expressions of toxicity.

YOUR BODY IS A DETOX MACHINE

Your health depends on your body's ability to eliminate toxins and waste from your cells, organs, and bloodstream. Healthy cells automatically detoxify themselves. Detoxification is a natural process that never stops in your body. Toxic materials and substances for which your body has no use are continually neutralized and eliminated. The process is so important that many interlocking and overlapping systems operate to accomplish this mission. Your body processes and expels chemicals and waste materials primarily through your skin, lungs, kidneys, liver, lymphatic system, and colon. These systems of elimination support and work together to keep you clean inside.

Some refer to a healthy body as a well-oiled, well-maintained machine that runs smoothly. Another way to look at the miracle of your body is to think of it as an orchestra. Each instrument has a distinct sound, and each musician an individual part to play. When all the players follow their music and play on key at the right tempo, the orchestra creates beautiful music. If members of the orchestra do not follow the music or the conductor, the piece falls apart and the sound is noise, not music. The same is true of your body. When the many systems work together in harmony and do what they are designed to do, you will feel great and enjoy excellent health. If the intricate balance of your body is overwhelmed by a toxic body burden, your health suffers. The good news is that you can restore the harmonious balance in your body by getting rid of the toxins that disrupt your bodily functions.

The Largest Organ of Elimination

Your skin is your largest organ of elimination. One way that toxins leave your body is through perspiration. It is a good idea to work up a sweat for twenty minutes three times a week after you have completed the detox. You have to make exercise part of your life during and after detoxing. Be sure to limit your exercise to no more than thirty minutes a day of gentle movement like walking or yoga during your detox month. Sauna, steam, and detox baths promote the excretion of heavy metals like lead, mercury, and cadmium and harmful fat-soluble chemicals like PCBs, PBBs, and HCBs, which we cover in more detail later.

The skin is also an organ of absorption. Putting something on your skin is like eating it. Think about the chemicals in soaps and lotions and permanent press clothing. What enters your body through your skin travels through your bloodstream and can damage cells before the chemicals reach your liver to be filtered out.

Deep Breathing

Polluted air causes asthma, bronchitis, and lung cancer. Studies have shown that parents who smoke increase the risk of their children developing asthma from their exposure to secondhand smoke. Even more disturbing, pollution is able to affect your DNA to produce genetic respiratory conditions in future generations. The contaminated air you breathe also affects your pH balance and can make your body acidic.

Your lungs filter the air, and your breath expels many contaminants when you exhale. The blood carries used and toxic gases to your lungs to be eliminated with each exhalation. When you sneeze or cough, you expel those toxins with force. If pollutants get stuck in your lungs, they enter your bloodstream and travel through your body causing damage, and can overwork other filtering systems.

Even taking a shower can be risky. The Environmental Protection Agency stated that a long, hot shower of ten minutes or more can be dangerous, because the chlorine in our water supply can evaporate into the air, forming a toxic gas that you inhale. Breathing that gas can increase your risk of bladder, kidney, and colon cancer. To remedy this, you can buy a showerhead that filters the water or have a filtration system on your main water line to avoid this health threat.

Breathing properly is an important part of detoxifying your body. You have to breathe deeply and fully to oxygenate your body and brain. Be aware when you are breathing only from the top portion of your lungs, and correct it. Poor posture compresses your lungs and restricts your breathing capacity, your oxygen uptake, and the elimination of toxic gases. Proper breathing helps keep lymphatic circulation moving to produce and deliver antibodies to fight off disease and to remove cellular waste.

Keep It Moving

Your body has two circulatory systems: the bloodstream and the lymphatic system. The pumping heart fuels the bloodstream, which moves cellular waste to the liver, kidneys, bladder, bowel, skin, and lungs for expulsion. Your bloodstream also delivers oxygen, nutrition, and hormones to the cells.

The lymphatic system, the other circulatory system, is a major component of the immune system. It helps the immune system by removing and destroying waste, debris, dead blood cells, pathogens, toxins, and cancer cells. It absorbs fat and fat-soluble vitamins from the digestive system and delivers these nutrients to the body's cells. The lymphatic system removes excess fluid and waste products from the spaces between the cells.

The lymphatic system does not have a heart to pump it. Its movement depends on the motions of the muscle and joints. As the lymph fluid moves upward toward the neck, it passes through the lymph nodes, which filter it to remove waste and pathogens. That is why lymphatic massage is helpful in removing toxins from your body.

The Major Processing Plant

The liver is a factory with more than 600 functions. It is a vital organ that responds to the demands of the body by shifting blood to specific areas. The liver stores blood sugar, which is called glycogen, and releases it into the bloodstream when it is needed. The liver signals the adrenal glands to regulate blood sugar. Insulin is one of the hormones regulated by the liver. Produced by the pancreas, insulin is required for your cells to absorb blood sugar to produce energy. The liver also controls fat metabolism and makes cholesterol.

The liver is a detox plant. It filters poisons in the bloodstream, neutralizes them, and sends them on to the elimination organs. When other organs are not functioning optimally, the liver becomes overloaded. The toxins pass through the liver a few times, damaging cells until the liver can neutralize the contaminants. This extra strain reduces the liver's ability to do other jobs. The results are high cholesterol, imbalanced hormones, unregulated blood sugar, and raised blood pressure. When the liver is overloaded, inflammation can result. If the liver is overwhelmed by excess toxins, they can be redeposited in the joints or as plaque on the walls of blood vessels and the intestines, held in cysts, or lodged in fatty areas of the brain, the breast, or the prostate.

> I lost thirty pounds right away and kept it off. I can't live without juicing and eating healthy every day now. It changed my life. Back in 2007, I was diagnosed with nonalcohol-related fatty liver disease. Since I did the diet detox last year, all my liver functions have returned to normal, along with a few other health issues I had. I owe my healthy living to this way of life now. I'm no doctor, but this detox diet has totally changed my life.
>
> M.B.

The liver can become a fat-storing organ if you do not eat well. A fatty liver results from a diet high in refined and fatty foods, sugar, high glycemic carbohydrates, some prescription medications, vitamin deficiencies, and alcohol consumption. Diabetes, high blood pressure, and obesity also tax this important organ.

The liver is a crucial target of the detox. A healthy liver will keep you clean inside. It is important to cleanse the liver before weight loss, because it will have to work overtime to filter the released toxins that have been stored in your fat cells. The next chapter explains how the storage of toxins in your fat cells makes you gain hard-to-lose weight.

The Kidneys and the Importance of Hydration

The kidneys filter and recirculate blood to flush out waste. They need plenty of water to do the job. The color of urine is the first sign of dehydration. A well-hydrated body produces urine that is mostly clear with only a slight tinge of yellow. If your urine has a strong odor or is dark in color, you are not drinking enough water.

More than 60 percent of your body is composed of water. Your brain is 70 percent water. The body needs pure water to operate healthfully. Water lubricates every process. Without enough of it, your cells cannot use nutrients for fuel, burn oxygen to give you energy, or generate the impulses in your nerves that make you move. Besides, being dehydrated ages you. You will not last more than three days without water. Your cells cannot function without it.

Dehydration can make you eat more. Aside from having a dry mouth, you can become hungry when your body needs water. You feel hunger because your body will get water from food. If your diet does not contain enough fruits and vegetables, which have high water content, you might develop salt cravings so that your body can retain water to operate smoothly. Then a sweet craving can kick in to compensate for the low energy that comes with dehydration.

When you hydrate, you do not want to consume water filled with toxic chemicals. Water is a vehicle for detoxing. What you drink should not contribute to your toxic load. For the detox, you will drink naturally distilled water.

Colon or Large Intestine

The colon receives solid waste from the rest of the body. Your large intestine, like your kidneys, needs to be properly hydrated and cleaned to work efficiently. When the colon is not doing its job, waste backs up into the bloodstream. To make up for the colon's inability to expel the toxins, the liver, skin, kidneys, and lungs have to work harder.

Solid waste accumulating in the colon suffocates cells by preventing nutrient absorption. The spaces around cells fill up with waste, which disrupts their normal function. Blood is not able to carry nutrients into the cells, and your body has difficulty building new cells. If the situation continues, cells and tissues will die. One way that affected cells struggle to survive is to expend a lot of energy in a last-ditch effort, reproducing very quickly. That uncontrolled production of new cells is called cancer.

When dead materials back up in the colon, high levels of bacteria, viruses, molds, and parasites feed on the waste matter, which they break down. The immune system moves in to help with elimination. Histamine is released to expel the waste, producing coughing, sneezing, a runny nose, and diarrhea. Your body becomes inflamed to kill off and remove the germs. That is your immune system at work. When your immune system is overwhelmed, disease sets in.

Poorly digested food limits the amount of nutrients available to be absorbed and increases your toxic burden. Carbohydrates ferment, protein putrefies, and fat becomes rancid, producing gases and toxic by-products that are reabsorbed and put stress on the body's elimination systems.

Keeping your colon clean and clear is a crucial element of good health. Along with drinking enough water, eating vegetables and fruit is crucial to bowel health. Fresh produce is a great source of fiber, which acts like a sponge for toxins. Fiber is not digested and passes through your stomach, small intestine, and large intestine and is eliminated intact. This bulk cleans out your colon as it moves through.

TOXIC LOAD AND THE "SOUP POT" THEORY

The unprecedented high level of toxins found in our environment has overwhelmed the body's ability to process and eliminate these poisons. Your body is not designed to process so many man-made chemicals, which build up. When those toxins accumulate, they damage your cells, interfere with your bodily functions, and compromise your well-being.

The term "toxic load" refers to all the contaminants in air, water, and food to which you have been exposed. Your emotions and stress also affect the mix. The accumulation of chemicals, toxins, and other substances that enter your body is called your body burden. Think of a pot of soup on the back burner of your stove. It will boil over if you add too many ingredients and cook it over too high a flame. Your body is like that pot. If it is loaded with toxins with the heat of too much stress, your body is not able to contain the toxic burden and will boil over. You might experience vague symptoms like headaches or dull hair. You might develop sensitivities and have allergic reactions. If you do not lower your body burden, you will get sick. Chronic health concerns are often the result of low-grade poisoning of your metabolism. A polluted environment, damaging lifestyle habits like smoking, drinking alcohol, eating processed food and conventionally grown produce, medications, and stress all contribute to your body burden.

There are many signs of toxic overload, including

Indigestion	Weak fingernails
Headaches	Fuzzy brain
Dull, brittle hair	Bad breath
Skin problems	Fatigue

Anxiety

Aggression

Depression

Stress sensitivity

Low energy

Lack of stamina

Allergies

Flatulence

Autoimmune diseases
like arthritis or
inflammatory bowel
disease

Cardiovascular disease

When toxins are stored in your body, they interrupt or completely block your metabolic functions. Your body's ability to move nutrients into cells, produce energy, make repairs, generate new cells, and process and eliminate waste is compromised. Your body becomes inflamed and acidic. Your immune system goes into overdrive, reacting constantly to the presence of toxins by trying to expel the foreign substances. This causes extreme stress to a system trying to protect you. Your body produces extra blood vessels to feed the growing toxic fat cells, which strains your heart. In an effort to dilute the circulating toxins, your body retains fluids. The systems described earlier in this chapter cannot accomplish what they have to do to keep you healthy. That is when nagging symptoms develop into full-fledged disease.

The good news is that you can stop this disintegration. You can enhance your body's natural ability to detox and begin to reverse the damage that has already been done by spending a month on the 1 Pound a Day Diet Detox. You can take action and accomplish a toxic reversal that lowers your body burden. We have seen it happen time and again. People come to the retreat in terrible shape and get their lives back. We have so many testimonials from people who have followed the simple program at home. Your body wants to heal itself. Why not do all you can to help? Every organ and system in your body will benefit from doing the detox presented in this book.

Two of the signs of impaired metabolism are weight gain and

difficulty losing weight. Recently, scientists have begun to speculate about the link between the dramatically increased exposure to environmental toxins during the last few decades and the obesity epidemic. The next chapter examines how toxins can make you gain weight and explains why detoxing helps you take it off.

Detox Success Story

CHANGING MY BODY FROM THE INSIDE OUT

I was overweight and had an ongoing battle with my weight over the course of several years. I heard Dr. Roni DeLuz talking about the Martha's Vineyard Diet Detox. It sounded like exactly what I needed, so I bought her book and read it cover to cover. I did the program and had great success. I learned a lot about my body and how my habits and even my thought processes can cause serious health problems.

In November 2011, I was diagnosed with cervical cancer. Four months later I had a radical hysterectomy. I needed to develop a plan and put it in motion. I knew that if I was going to live a long time and live healthy, I would have to turn my life 180 degrees. I decided to do the detox again. This time I wanted more than a quick weight-loss plan. I needed to change my body from the inside out if I wanted to be truly healthy and to remain cancer-free.

A friend recommended the movie *Fat, Sick, and Nearly Dead*. Watching that movie was eye-opening. After learning about the damage that toxins in processed foods, chemicals, and environmental sources can do to the body and the illnesses they can cause, I was determined to do a diet detox to rid my body of these toxins and loosen up some of the fat cells that stored them. A detox works with the body to do the job it can't do itself—get rid of the toxins and flush out fat cells.

In July 2012, I started a sixty-day detox to rid my body of built-up toxins. I went from a size 18 to a size 10 in pants. I feel better than I ever have. My husband did the detox as well. He is an over-the-road trucker who lives on the road for months at a time. He managed to stick with it all sixty days. Juicing will always be part of a healthy diet for me. Knowing that I could be dealing with a life-threatening illness keeps me focused on my health, and I will do whatever I can to keep my body healthy and toxin-free.

The program really works. I attribute my cancer not spreading to Dr. Roni's detox.

Heather Smith

CHAPTER 2

⤳

EASY TO GAIN, HARD TO LOSE

If you are having problems with your weight, you are not alone. More than two-thirds of adults in the United States are overweight and nearly one-third are obese. Nearly one in three children and teenagers is overweight. To put these figures in another perspective, from 1980 to 2008 the rates of obesity have doubled for adults and tripled for children. The concern is global. For the first time in history, more people will die of diseases linked to obesity and subsequent metabolic dysfunction than starvation or malnutrition. The supersizing of the American diet, fast and processed foods, and our sedentary lifestyle had been considered the major contributors to the obesity epidemic. But overeating and inactivity cannot completely account for the epidemic rise in obesity during the past three decades. This alarming trend involves more than just an individual's lifestyle or willpower.

As we have said before, the increased production and use of synthetic chemicals during the past forty to fifty years have changed the environment drastically. The fattening of America has paralleled our increased exposure to contaminants. Evidence has emerged pointing to a link between toxins and obesity. Scientists are speculating that the current level of our chemical exposure may have damaged many of the body's natural weight-control mechanisms.

TOXINS AND FAT

When you carry toxins, excess stress hormones, and inflammation, your body tries to protect you. When a toxic overload accumulates, your biochemistry begins to shift to fat production. Fat acts as a protective buffer for toxins. When toxins are not effectively processed by the liver and eliminated, the body keeps them from circulating in the bloodstream by storing some of them in fat, creating a toxic dump, particularly around your middle. This is a form of self-defense against being poisoned. When you reduce your toxic load, your body shifts away from fat production.

Many toxic chemicals are fat-soluble. These toxins are stored in fat cells to get the poisons out of circulation and away from key organs. Water-soluble toxins are more easily eliminated through your sweat glands and urinary system. The fat-soluble toxins that are stored in your cells can disrupt the hormone signaling system that controls your appetite and metabolism. The toxins increase inflammation. They can reprogram cells to become new fat cells. The newly formed cells may not be able to create energy efficiently. Those cells fill with excess fat and even more toxins that are not being metabolized. You just keep gaining weight.

> Before I did this diet the first time, I took a pill at the drop of a hat. I took pills for every little thing. I was on a drug called Soma and coming off it was a very bad trip. I lost twenty-five pounds in twenty-one days and a total of sixty. I went from a size 16 to a size 6. I could not have jump-started my weight loss any other way.
>
> Now I am training for a triathlon. I have so much energy, and have become a vegan. I feel wonderful and wish I could have felt this good in my thirties. I am now forty-three and feel thirty-three.
>
> S.H.

The toxins in your fat cells can trigger the release of leptin, a hormone that tells the brain about the changes in the amount of fat tissue that is in the body and regulates appetite. If leptin levels stay too highly elevated for too long, leptin receptors can burn out, leading to a condition known as leptin resistance. The "burn fat" message is not transmitted. When this happens, you are hungrier, are likely to eat more, and continue to gain weight that is hard to shed.

TOXINS THAT MESS WITH YOUR HORMONES

The hormones in your body are chemical messengers that communicate between your organs, your brain, and the environment. Disrupting this communication can result in serious health consequences. There is a class of synthetic chemicals called endocrine disrupters. These chemicals interfere with the production of hormones and how they do their jobs. Some hormone disrupters actually mimic hormones, particularly estrogen, tricking your body by interfering with communication between the brain and other vital organs. Aside from fat accumulation, hormone disrupters affect you in many other ways, resulting in:

Low energy
Slowed metabolism
Muscle loss
Mood disorders
Low sex drive
Thyroid problems
Immune disorders
Early puberty
Breast development in boys

As you can see, toxins that disrupt your hormones can have a devastating effect on the quality of your life. Even more disturbing, endocrine disrupters can affect the hormone signaling pathways of babies growing in the womb and newborns during critical stages of development. The effects are often not apparent until much later in life. Scientists suspect that this action has been contributing to the childhood obesity epidemic.

OBESOGENS AND WEIGHT GAIN

Even low exposure to certain toxins can seriously disrupt your metabolism. Scientists have recently discovered a class of toxins identified as "obesogens" that disrupt the regulation of fat storage and energy balance. These toxins change the systems that control your weight by increasing the number of fat cells you have, decreasing the calories you burn, and changing the way your body manages hunger.

Let's take a look at a few of these obesogens and where you are likely to come into contact with them.

Nicotine: If a mother smokes during pregnancy, her baby has a higher risk of becoming overweight or obese later in life than if the mother does not smoke during pregnancy.

High fructose corn syrup is an ingredient in most processed foods. It contributes to insulin resistance and interferes with leptin appetite control. Consuming corn syrup creates a weight-gain cycle: you crave more food that is quickly stored as fat.

BPA (bisphenol A) is used to make plastic hard. It is found in plastic bottles, can linings, thermal paper used for cash register receipts, and household electronics. The chemical has been found in 93 percent of Americans tested. BPA increases insulin resistance, which lowers energy production and leads to diabetes. BPA has been linked to obesity, developmental delays in children, and thyroid problems.

PFOA (perfluorooctanoic acid) is a component of nonstick coatings of pots and pans, the lining of microwave popcorn bags, and finishes on stain-resistant fabrics. This compound affects the thyroid hormones.

Phthalates, which are plasticizers, are hard to avoid. They are commonly found in toys, cosmetics, cleaning products, air fresheners, shower curtains, perfume, vinyl flooring, plastic food containers, and commercial food packaging. Phthalates have been associated with weight gain and loss of muscle mass.

Pesticides and herbicides are sprayed on conventionally grown crops. They enter the cells of plants we consume, leach into the soil, and run off into our water supply. Some insecticides and herbicides are found in the grain fed to livestock, where they are stored in animal fat. When you consume meat, poultry, and farm-raised fish that have been fed treated grains, the pesticides are stored in your fat cells.

Hormones and antibiotics used to fatten livestock accumulate in the animals' fat cells and are passed on to you when you eat conventionally raised beef, pork, and poultry. The role of these chemicals is to slow down the metabolism of the animals so that they gain weight. When you eat meat or poultry that has been treated with these chemicals, your body responds the same way. The chemicals fatten you up.

We have mentioned only a few of the known obesogens. As research continues in this new field, scientists are bound to find hundreds if not thousands more chemicals that are associated with the obesity epidemic. We are being supersized by more than the portions we eat and our food choices. If you want to stay healthy, detoxing is a necessity, not a choice.

DETOX WILL HELP YOU BREAK THROUGH WEIGHT PLATEAUS

Toxins stored in fat cells can remain stuck there. It is hard to lose toxic fat. Your body resists releasing these toxins. When you lose weight, fat cells are burned to create energy. As fat cells are metabolized, stored toxins are released back into circulation. The freed-up toxins lower your thyroid hormone levels, which slows down your metabolic rate and curtails fat burning. The more fat you start with,

Twenty Ways to Avoid Obesogens

Obesogens enter your body from what you eat and drink, from chemicals and dust in the air that you breathe, and through your skin from the cosmetics and household cleaners you use. You do not live in a bubble. Living in the modern world makes exposure to these toxins inescapable, but you can take steps to reduce your exposure. Every little bit helps. Here are some changes you can make that will protect you and your family.

1. Eat organic produce.
2. Eat meat and poultry that has been raised without hormones or antibiotics. Grass-fed beef and free-range poultry are good choices.
3. Eat wild fish, not farmed.
4. Reduce your consumption of animal fats, which are high in stored toxins. A high-fat diet can intensify the effects of obesogens.
5. Minimize the amount of processed foods you eat.
6. Stay away from high fructose corn syrup.
7. Limit your consumption of soy products. Despite having high levels of protein, soy promotes fat-cell growth because of its plant-based estrogen properties.
8. Eat fresh or frozen food rather than canned.
9. Use a filter on the faucet in your kitchen and the showerhead, or have a filter installed on the central water line. At the very least, filter your drinking water.
10. Avoid using nonstick pans, especially if they are scratched.
11. Do not use plastic food containers for leftovers. Discard any plastics with a 3 or 7 on the bottom. Glass is best.
12. Ask your grocer to wrap your meat, poultry, and seafood in paper, not plastic.
13. Do not use plastic or Styrofoam cups.
14. Use only BPA-free, ecofriendly water bottles. Stainless-steel or glass bottles are best.
15. Never microwave plastic.
16. Open your windows to ventilate your home. Do not use air fresheners.

17. Replace vinyl shower curtains with cloth. The heat from a shower will cause chemicals to outgas, and you will inhale the gases in the mist.
18. Use an exhaust fan when cooking.
19. Vacuum frequently with a HEPA-filtered vacuum cleaner.
20. Minimize your exposure to thermal paper used for cash register receipts. Make sure to wash your hands after handling receipts.

Your detox will be more effective and longer lasting if you incorporate some or all of these changes into your life. You will also boost your ability to lose weight and keep it off.

the more toxins are released. Your body wants to store those toxins as fat, making it difficult to lose additional weight. In other words, weight loss prevents further weight loss. That is why diets do not work.

The way to break this frustrating cycle is to detox, which will put your systems of elimination in good working order. Only then will your body be able to flush out the toxins weight loss releases. The 1 Pound a Day Diet Detox achieves this on a cellular level. The toxins trapped in your cells will be set free and flushed out of your body. This will reduce your fat cells. We always say that weight loss is a by-product of detoxing. Now you understand why.

Detox Success Story
I DON'T WANT TO WEAR MY FOOD

Growing up, I was an underweight kid. I ate only as much as I needed to feel full and played outside all the time. It was not until I married in my twenties that my thyroid went berserk. I had the onset of Graves' disease and enough TSH [thyroid-stimulating hormone] in my body for four people. I had hyperthyroidism. As a result, my heart was accelerating. Tests showed that my heart was perfect, just beating rapidly. Then my doctor discovered the culprit in the blood tests. He put me on a small dose of beta blocker to calm my beating heart. His thinking was that my body would correct the thyroid. It did, but I gained eighty pounds within six months. Not good on my five-foot, five-inch frame. I had stretch marks and no babies to show for them.

I cried in my doctor's office. He explained that he knew I would not take the beta blocker if he told me I could gain weight. I needed to take that medication to slow down my heart, so he did not tell me about that particular side effect. This started my yo-yo dieting that continued to 2008.

I went through a divorce in 2002 and controlled my weight and anger with running. Forgiveness came, but I pulled my ACL in 2007 and put on weight. I was a size 4/6 top and 12/14 bottom. I did the Martha's Vineyard Diet Detox in March 2008 and lost twenty-two pounds. My pants size went down to an 8/10. I had not seen that size since college and my twenties.

I am an emotional eater and a lot has been going on in my life, so here we are in 2012, and I've regained. I'm wearing my food again, but I know what I need to do to get on track. My body responds best to juicing and the Martha's Vineyard Diet Detox. I'm taking my health back once again. I can taste the veggie juice now!

Kimberly Kirkland Absher

CHAPTER 3

～

THE BEST DEFENSE

Now that you know how toxins are hurting you, you should be fired up to do something about it. Your body never stops working to defend you from harm. Your cells fight for survival. All the systems in your body work to restore the balance that toxins disrupt. Unless you give your body some relief, it will break down.

If you want to lighten your toxic load, you have to do three things:

1. You have to be aware of the toxins around you and do whatever you can to avoid or decrease your exposure.
2. You have to support your body to process toxic substances.
3. You have to bolster the elimination mechanisms.

The best way to achieve these goals is to do the 1 Pound a Day Diet Detox. The detox will restore your body's equilibrium by helping it rid itself of toxins, while resting your digestive system at the same time. When you detoxify, your vital organs get a rest so that your energy can go toward healing. Tired and abused organs need a break to repair themselves. Our detox draws out waste on a cellular level in preparation for a healthier rebuilding. The detox provides maximum nutrition for cleansing and healing.

WHY THE 1 POUND A DAY DIET DETOX IS MORE EFFECTIVE THAN FASTING OR JUICE CLEANSES

The grandfather of all fasting cleanses is the Master Cleanse. The regimen involves drinking water with lemon juice, maple syrup, and cayenne pepper. That's it. The nutritional value of the drink is obviously minimal. Of course you will lose weight if that drink is all you consume. Your digestive organs definitely will get a rest—you are consuming very little that needs to be digested. The minute you start eating again, the pounds will come right back, and more. If you stay on the Master Cleanse, your body will go into starvation mode and your metabolism will slow down. You will hit the wall, reach a weight plateau, and probably get sick. You can also lose muscle mass, which you do not want to happen, because muscles consume a lot of energy and burn calories. Without proper nutrients, the body will begin to break down cells in muscle tissue for energy.

Juice fasts or cleanses are all the rage now. You can buy fresh-squeezed bottled juices everywhere. There are juice carts on the streets of New York. Starbucks is about to sell its own brand of health juices. Even supermarkets sell bottled vegetable juices.

Many prepared juices are made with sweet fruits and vegetables to make the juices palatable. Sweet juices raise your blood sugar and stimulate insulin production. Your pancreas has to churn out so much insulin it can become tired and sluggish. Too much insulin can lead to insulin resistance, which drives metabolic diseases like type 2 diabetes, hypertension, heart disease, and fatty liver disease. The sugar from the juice is rapidly absorbed into the bloodstream, and the liver processes it for energy use. The purpose of doing a cleanse is to give your organs a rest. Juices that are sweet will prevent this from happening. Once again, you will lose weight, because your caloric intake is so low.

> Only your body can heal you. You have to give it the support it needs when you have robbed it of nutrition for years.
>
> Robin Quivers

When you are on a juice cleanse, your diet is limited to fresh vegetable and fruit juices and water, usually for three to ten days. These cleanses can result in the loss of muscle tissue and good bacteria in your digestive system. Cleansing for a few days does rid your body of some toxins, but the detoxification is not as profound as the results of our program. The 1 Pound a Day Diet Detox is a total body cleanse that detoxifies all the organs of elimination—the skin, lungs, kidneys, liver, lymphatic system, and colon.

Another problem with juice fasts is that when vegetables and fruits are juiced, the fiber content is left behind in the juicer. Fiber is essential for cleaning out your colon and absorbing toxins. Juice cleanses might jump-start weight loss, just as the Master Cleanse does, but you will put the weight right back on when you return to your normal eating habits.

The detox you are about to begin provides your body with very high quality nutrition in small doses. You will be taking additional supplements that are not a part of other cleanses. Taking the supplements we recommend is essential if you want to cleanse your body deeply. You will be bathing your cells in pure, easily digested nutrients every two hours. A well-nourished body will start to release stored toxins from fat cells. Your fat cells will shrink, and you will lose inches and weight. Since you are not depriving your body of nutrition, you will avoid the frustrating yo-yo effect once you are off the detox program. The soup you eat every night will provide fiber, which helps your body eliminate toxins. Fiber also makes you feel full. You will take a supplement to support the enzymes to ease digestion, make the process more efficient, and reduce the demands on your organs. *1 Pound a Day* takes care to correct the shortcomings of other cleanses and juice fasts. That is why our detox is so effective.

Another important difference is expense. The cleanses available today cost between fifty and a hundred dollars a day, beyond the reach of most people. Our detox will run you fifteen dollars a day, and that includes the supplements. Fifteen dollars is a small investment for the return you will receive. You probably spend more than that on coffee, soft drinks, snacks, take-out, or fast food every day. And none of that food is good for you.

THE THREE LEVELS OF FOOD

No matter how careful you are, you cannot live in this world without being exposed to toxins. The previous chapter gave you suggestions for some simple changes you can make in your environment to reduce your toxic load. Making adjustments in how you nourish your body is the single most important thing you can do to be healthy, lose toxic fat, and restore your energy. You have complete control over the food you eat. You make a choice every time you put something in your mouth.

Our goal in this book is to help you transform yourself by changing your eating habits. We want to convince you to make the shift from what we call overcivilized food to fresh and organic food accompanied by high-density nutritional supplements. Those three categories of food form a chain that progresses from food that makes you sick to a way of eating that will support your health, maintain weight loss, and finally heal and rejuvenate. There are many benefits to moving up that chain.

Level One: Overcivilized Food

We consider the lowest level of food "overcivilized" because it is so highly refined. The processed foods that fill supermarkets are very far removed from their natural state. These colorfully packaged convenience foods have had the life processed out of them. If food is canned, jarred, bagged, or boxed with a list of ingredients on the label, consider it processed.

To begin with, processed foods are usually manufactured with heavily refined, processed ingredients like white flour, which has had almost all of its nutrition ground away during the milling process, leaving only empty calories. These dead processed foods have been stripped of nutrients during processing, then "enriched" with synthetic vitamins and minerals. Other chemicals are added to make them look better and last longer. Ingredients are added to processed foods to stabilize, emulsify, texturize, soften, preserve, sweeten, deodorize, bleach, and color. These additives can be highly toxic. Some of them are downright disgusting. Take the pink slime scandal.

Pink slime—also known as "lean finely textured beef," "mechanically separated meat," and "boneless beef lean trimmings"—is a filler used by meat processors. They grind up scraps and meat trimmings and add ammonia gas to disinfect the ground meat. The trimmings used in pink slime are full of infectious agents or pathogens before they are treated. Manufacturers use ammonia in gas form to kill off the pathogens to keep people from getting sick from eating pink slime. That is the same poisonous ammonia found in liquid form in most cleaning products. Let us repeat: Meat processors take meat that is too dangerous to feed humans and disinfect it with a highly toxic substance.

Seventy percent of supermarket ground beef contains pink slime. Though McDonald's, Taco Bell, and Burger King have phased out this additive, it is a staple of food served in school cafeterias. Does that make any sense to you? Think twice and read labels before you buy or order hot dogs, lunch meat, chili, sausages, pepperoni, canned meats, and frozen entrées, unless you want to risk being slimed.

Aside from being nutrient-deficient, heavily processed foods promote unhealthy weight gain and obesity, because they are usually high in sugar, trans fats, and salt, and low in fiber. Overrefined foods sabotage staying at a healthy weight in another, more insidious way. Processed foods are created to have strong flavors. Once you are used to the excessive sugar, salt, and MSG found in convenience foods, your taste buds are affected. Your natural sense of taste is destroyed. You become a high-flavor addict. You no longer taste the subtleties of natural flavors in whole foods. You want to add salt or sugar to everything. How often have you seen people pouring salt on their food before they have even tasted it? Too much salt or sugar is definitely not good for your weight and your health.

FOOD ADDITIVE ALERT

The Food and Drug Administration has a list of more than 3,000 substances that can be added to foods for the purpose of preservation, coloring, texture, flavor enhancement, and more. Most have never been tested, but some are known to be dangerous. These additives can cause allergies, genetic mutations, and cancer, to name just a few negative health effects. Being aware of the chemicals hidden in processed food should make eating them a lot less appealing. Your body pays a high price for convenience. Knowing more about these dangerous ingredients will motivate you to choose healthy foods. We want to

> As a nation, we are clueless about preservatives and additives and how they are literally killing us. Your book should be a must-read in school to turn our society around about what truly is good. Detox, detox, detox . . . Do it the Martha's Vineyard way. Get the bad stuff out and then feed your body with good, healthy food. This detox changed me in the most positive way.
>
> S.L.

give you a brief survey of the worst of the worst food additives, so you will know them when you see them.

Artificial Sweeteners Can Make You Fat

Though artificial sweeteners contain no calories, they can contribute to weight problems and make you fat. The body judges the number of calories in food by how it tastes. Sugar substitutes separate the taste of sweetness from the calories. When you drink a diet soda, your taste buds communicate to your brain that energy is coming in, but your body does not get the fuel it expects. Artificial sweeteners can upset your food chemistry and interfere with your body's natural regulating processes.

They trick your body in another way. Artificial sweeteners are 200 to 13,000 times as sweet as sugar. The "feel good" hormones in your brain, called endorphins, respond to such an extremely strong sweet signal. As endorphin levels are boosted, your pleasure increases. Studies have shown that this elevation can lead to eating more. The taste of sweetness is mildly addictive. The more sweets you eat, the more you need to feel satisfied. Someone at the retreat once said to us, "Thin people don't drink diet cola." It has to do with more than calories.

The artificial sweeteners to look out for are:

Aspartame is used in more than 9,000 food products, including NutraSweet and Equal. It is found in diet and sugar-free sodas and drinks, yogurt, breath mints, instant breakfasts, and frozen desserts. The body breaks down aspartame into the toxic by-products formic acid and formaldehyde, a powerful neurotoxin and carcinogen. This sugar substitute breaks down at temperatures of 86°F and above, so it should never be used in hot drinks or for cooking. Aspartame has been linked to migraines, memory loss, seizures, Parkinson's disease, and brain tumors. It accounts for more reports to the Food and Drug Administration than all other foods and food additives combined.

Saccharin: This sugar substitute is used in Sweet 'N Low. It can cause bladder cancer and has been tied to weight gain. The Food and Drug Administration recommended that it be banned from use. The government responded by putting a warning label on the product.

Acesulfame K: This sweetener is used in baked goods, chewing gum, and soft drinks. It was approved by the Food and Drug Administration in 1988, but there have been no long-term studies of the sweetener. It contains the carcinogen methylene chloride. This artificial sweetener has been linked to headaches, depression, nausea, liver, kidney, and thyroid probems as well.

MSG (monosodium glutamate)

If you eat take-out Chinese food, you may have experienced some of the side effects of MSG: the headaches, bloat, and sluggishness that typically follow the meal. MSG is an amino acid that is used as a flavor enhancer in almost all processed foods and fast foods, and by most chain restaurants. The skin of Kentucky Fried Chicken is full of MSG. You will find it in flavored chips, salad dressings, frozen dinners, sausages, hot dogs, canned tuna, protein powders, and instant foods like soups.

Knowing that people want to avoid MSG, manufacturers often hide its presence on the label by making it a part of another ingredient. MSG goes by many names on labels. Look out for gelatin, glutamate, hydrolyzed protein, yeast extract, textured protein, hydrolyzed vegetable protein, hydrolyzed plant protein, vegetable protein extract, glutamic acid, sodium caseinate, soy protein isolates, barley malt, calcium caseinate, and malt extract.

This ubiquitous flavor enhancer is neurotoxic, meaning it can cause neurons to die. MSG is used in laboratories to induce obesity in rats for experiments. It acts in the same way in our bodies. In addition to obesity, it can lead to type 2 diabetes and metabolic syndrome.

Food Coloring

Food colorings are made from coal tar and petrochemicals. How unappetizing could an ingredient be? Some food colorings are carcinogenic and can affect enzymes. The European Union has labeling regulations for informing consumers of the health risks of these additives, but the United States does not.

Food coloring is used in energy bars, cereal, beverages, candy, baked goods, jams, macaroni and cheese, deli meats, puddings, condiments, ice cream, sherbet, fast food. They are also used on meat and fish to make them appear fresher. There are seven colorings for which you should be on the lookout:

Red #3 is what gives the maraschino cherries in canned fruit salad such intense color. It has caused thyroid cancer in animal studies. The Food and Drug Administration advised that this food coloring be removed from the market, but the recommendation was overruled.

Red #40 has done damage to the liver, colon, and stomach in animal studies. It is suspected to be a carcinogen. Some children may be sensitive to this additive, which has been found to increase behavior issues, hyperactivity, and attention problems.

Blue #1 is a skin and eye irritant and an allergen. You will find it in beverages, candy, and baked goods.

Blue #2 has caused brain tumors in animal studies. It is an ingredient in pet food, candy, and beverages.

Yellow #6 has been linked to skin irritations, asthmatic reactions, adrenal gland and kidney tumors, and hyperactivity in children. It is used to color sausages, gelatin, candy, and baked goods.

Green #3 has caused tumors in animal studies. There is some controversy about this food coloring. More studies have to be done.

Caramel coloring is produced by heating sugars. Sometimes ammonia is used in the process, and toxic by-products are created. Those chemicals have been linked to cancer. Food companies are not required to reveal if they made the coloring with ammonia, so you do not know what you are consuming. Caramel coloring is used in colas, sauces, breads, and pastries.

BHA (Butylated Hydroxyanisole) and BHT (Butylated Hydroxytoluene)
These petroleum-derived chemicals are used as preservatives to keep fats and oils from going rancid. They are widely used to extend the shelf life of processed foods. The preservatives are found in cereals, chewing gum, vegetable oil, potato chips and other snack foods, butter, meats, and even beer. Scientists think the chemicals might change as they preserve food to form a compound that reacts in the body.

BHA is a known carcinogen. BHT is less dangerous but has resulted in cancer in some animal studies. The negative effects on humans include hyperactivity, asthma, skin problems, and disruption of estrogen balance.

Propyl Gallate
This preservative, thought to be carcinogenic, is often used with BHA and BHT to prevent fats and oils from spoiling. It can be found in chicken soup base, chewing gum, and vegetable oil.

Sodium Nitrate and Nitrite
These chemicals are added to meats to stabilize them and to give them their red color. These preservatives extend the life of meats and prevent the growth of bacteria. In your stomach they form nitrosamines, chemical compounds that are very strong carcinogens. They have been associated with liver disorders as well. Manufacturers have begun to add acids to meat treated with nitrates and nitrites to slow down the formation of nitrosamines. This has reduced the harm but not eliminated it entirely. Unless the products are otherwise labeled, you will find nitrates and nitrites in lunch meat, corned beef, smoked fish, hot dogs, and bacon—even turkey bacon.

Trans Fats (Hydrogenated and Partially Hydrogenated Oils)
Trans fats are made when hydrogen gas reacts with oil. The process is used to reduce cost and increase the stability and shelf life of food. Eating these fats, which are hard to avoid in processed food,

can lead to heart disease and diabetes. Trans fats involve a higher risk of heart disease than saturated fats, found in butter, cheese, and beef. Trans fats raise total cholesterol levels and deplete HDL, the good cholesterol that protects against heart disease. Margarine, vegetable shortening, crackers, cookies, baked goods, salad dressings, bread, chips, icing, and microwave popcorn all contain trans fats.

Olestra

Olestra is a zero-calorie fat substitute that is used to make fat-free potato chips and other baked and fried snacks. Our enzymes cannot digest olestra. It passes through the intestine intact, causing many digestive problems like stomach cramps, bloating, flatulence, and diarrhea. It inhibits the absorption of some important nutrients. Olestra binds with fat-soluble vitamins A, E, D, and K and beta-carotene, which normally function to keep the immune system healthy and to prevent some cancers.

Potassium Bromate

This oxidizing agent is used in making bread and rolls to increase volume. Animal studies have proved it to be highly carcinogenic. This additive has been associated with tumors in the kidney and thyroid gland. The European Union, Canada, and several other countries have banned its use. California requires a cancer warning on the label. Potassium bromate can also be called bromic acid, potassium salt, bromated flour, and "enriched flour" on labels.

High Fructose Corn Syrup (HFCS)

This is a highly refined sweetener made by separating cornstarch from the corn kernel, then converting the cornstarch to syrup. Nearly all HFCS is made from genetically modified corn. We will discuss the significance of this in a later section. Food manufacturers use HFCS as an inexpensive alternative to cane and beet sugar in thousands of products. The number one source of calories in the standard American diet, HFCS is the most common sweetener found in processed foods and beverages. It sustains freshness in baked goods and maintains sweetness in a beverage. HFCS is used to sweeten salad dressings, ketchup, cereal, soda, yogurt, soups, lunch meats, condiments, and candy, to name just a few food items. Americans unknowingly consume twelve teaspoons of HFCS a day on average. Look for these aliases on labels: corn sugar, glucose/fructose syrup, high-fructose maize syrup, insulin, isoglucose, and fruit fructose.

Some scientists have speculated that HFCS predisposes the body to turn fructose—or sugar—into fat. Obesity rates have skyrocketed since the introduction of HFCS thirty years ago. Researchers have found mercury, a toxic heavy metal, in nine of twenty samples of commercial HFCS.

Although HFCS has been demonized lately, it is very close to being identical to table sugar. The problem is that we are consuming more sugar of every sort in processed food. Obesity rates have gone up as our food supply and eating habits have changed. We are overdosing on sugar.

White Sugar (Sucrose)
According to the Department of Agriculture, Americans on average consume 156 pounds of sugar a year (more than thirty-one five-pound bags), much of it from processed foods. No wonder there is an obesity epidemic.

All the vitamins, minerals, proteins, enzymes, and other nutrients are stripped away when sugarcane or sugar beets are refined to produce pure sucrose. Table sugar is a concentrated, unnatural substance that is difficult for your body to handle, particularly when you eat excessive quantities. Sugar causes a rapid spike in your blood sugar. The body stops burning fat as fuel because the elevated blood sugar level signals that enough energy is available. Your metabolism slows down and your weight goes up.

Sugar causes diabetes and both hyperglycemia and hypoglycemia. Sugar consumption has been linked to heart disease, arteriosclerosis, hypertension, mental illness, depression, senility, and cancer.

* * *

We have focused on the most commonly used additives, but this brief list should give you an idea of just how tainted processed food is. Our advice is to avoid the center aisles of the supermarket and to stick to the outer aisles where the fresh food is sold. The reason fresh food is located on the perimeter is that those departments have to be restocked more often, because shelf life is short with fresh food. When it comes to additives, follow this simple rule: never buy food that contains ingredients you cannot pronounce. Now that you are about to shop the outer rim of the supermarket, you are ready to move to the second level of the food chain: fresh, clean, and green.

Level Two: Fresh, Organic, Whole Foods

We live in a land of plenty, but most of us are nutritionally deficient. We are starved for nourishment. The acronym for the standard American diet is SAD, which could not be more appropriate.

A statistical look at our eating habits underscores how badly we eat:

- 1 in 4 Americans eats fast food every day.
- 20 percent of meals are eaten in the car.
- About 1 in 4 eats more than 2 servings of vegetables a day.
- Less than 1 in 3 has more than 1 serving of fruit a day.
- In 2000, we consumed an average of 57 more pounds of meat than our annual average in the 1950s.
- In 2000, we ate the equivalent of 52 teaspoons of sugar a day.

Almost all of us can stand to improve the way we eat. You are now informed about the health risks that come with eating processed food. Your month-long detox will start you on the right path to nourishing yourself with whole foods as Nature made them. Fresh foods are far less toxic than the overcivilized foods of Level One. Your food cravings will disappear and so will your hunger.

CONVENTIONAL VERSUS ORGANIC PRODUCE

There has been a long-standing controversy about the benefits of buying organic fruits and vegetables. Stanford University published a study in September 2012 that made headlines and had the blogosphere buzzing. Analyzing 237 studies of organic produce and meats that met research criteria, the meta-analysis concluded that organic foods are no more nutritious than those that are conventionally produced. In support of the nutritional value of organic food, some have argued that since fewer poisons are used to farm organically, there are more nutrients in the soil that could raise the nutritional content of the produce.

> Those poisons we carry around in our body start to break us down like termites in a house. By choosing the right foods and exercising, we can keep them at bay.
>
> Phyllis Jennings

Though studies exist that have found organic food to be more nutritious, this is not the only reason people buy organic food. First, organic food is more flavorful, because livestock and produce are allowed to mature naturally. People often choose to pay more for organic produce to avoid the harmful pesticides, hormones, and other chemicals used by conventional agriculture. The environmental effects of conventional farming practices on the planet and animal welfare are other concerns.

Conventional farming uses chemical fertilizers; organically grown food is fertilized with manure, compost, or other natural substances to enrich the soil and feed the plants. More than 400 chemical pesticides are routinely used in conventional farming. These pesticides are endocrine disrupters. Residues remain on conventional food even after washing. Pesticides used in conventional farming linger in your body and remain long after you eat. Organic farmers use only natural pesticides or bugs and birds to control the pests. When it comes to weeds, you guessed it—synthetic herbicides are used in conventional agriculture; organic farmers rotate crops, till, and mulch to take care of weeds. In short, organic farming practices take care of the planet, reducing pollution and encouraging soil and water conservation. Conventional agriculture robs our food of more than sixty natural and vital trace elements. Conventional farming poisons our food supply, the air we breathe, the water we drink, and the soil in which crops are grown. Those should be enough reasons to convince you to buy organic produce.

It used to be that you had to search in health food stores to find organic products. Now so many people are conscious of the benefits that you can find organic produce even in the big box stores. From 1997 to 2011—just fourteen years—sales of organic foods increased from $3.6 billion to $24.4 billion. Eating organic is more expensive, but consider the cost to your family's health and the health of the environment of not buying organic produce and meat.

> For the detox, you should try to buy only organically produced vegetables. You do not want to introduce new toxins to replace the ones you are flushing out.

The "locavore" movement has spurred the founding of local farmers' markets all over the country. Shopping at your local market will reduce the carbon footprint of the food you eat, because it does not have to be shipped long distances. You will be supporting local farmers, and the very fresh food you buy is usually less expensive. To find a farmers' market near you, check www.localharvest.org.

THE NEW THREAT: GENETICALLY MODIFIED FOOD

Genetic engineers have been experimenting with our food supply. They are creating genetically modified organisms (GMOs) by moving genes from the DNA of one organism to another. They extract specific genes from one organism and force those genes into the DNA of another. The genes that are transferred can come from viruses, bacteria, insects, animals, and even humans.

This technique is used on crop plants to be eaten by animals and humans. The plants are modified to enhance desired traits. Genetic engineering can create plants with exactly the desired characteristics very quickly. Qualities the researchers are working on include pest resistance, herbicide tolerance (so that weeds can be killed chemically without injuring the crop), disease resistance, cold tolerance, drought tolerance, and nutritional enrichment.

Genetically modified food first appeared in the food supply in 1990. The current commercialized GMO crops include:

94 percent of soy
90 percent of canola
95 percent of sugar beets

These crops and their derivatives are widely used in processed food. Tomatoes and cantaloupes have been created with modified ripening. GMOs can trick consumers about the freshness of products. A beautiful red, ripe genetically modified tomato could be weeks old. Soybeans and sugar beets have been made resistant to herbicides. Corn and cotton plants now have increased resistance to pests. All of this sounds good, but there is a downside.

Genetically modified crops have been banned as food ingredients in Europe and elsewhere. The Food and Drug Administration (FDA) in the United States does not even require labeling. These foods constitute one-fourth of our food supply. Without labeling, there is no way to know which foods contain GMOs. Proposition 37, an initiative to establish mandatory labeling of genetically engineered food, was on the November 6, 2012, ballot in California, where it was defeated.

Genetically modified foods been linked to toxic and allergic reactions, sterility, sickness, and even death in livestock. Animal laboratory studies have found damage to every organ. To date, the effects on humans of consuming these modified foods have not been studied. Genetically engineered foods have not been around long enough for the risks to be known.

Genetically altered food can expose humans to toxins and allergens that have never been seen before. In 1989, this happened with the supplement L-tryptophan. The bacteria in the supplement were altered, and a new and toxic substance was produced. More than 1,500 people got sick from the supplement, and thirty-seven died. No one knows about how GMOs interact. Genetically modified foods or medications could interact to produce negative reactions. The crops have not been in our food supply long enough for us to know.

Plants genetically engineered to resist herbicides will increase the amount of herbicide used. Since their crops can tolerate the herbicides, farmers will use them more liberally. Crops grown from genetically modified seeds can affect neighboring weeds, which become resistant to herbicides. When this happens, more chemicals are needed to kill weeds, and those chemicals poison the soil, water, and food supply. The same thing happens with pesticides. When foods are altered to minimize the need for pesticides, insects will become resistant to commonly used pesticides over time. This could produce a real insect problem that threatens crops. Genetically engineered crops manufacture their own pesticides, increasing the pesticides in our food and land.

Early on, scientists thought modified genes were destroyed during the process of digestion. Recent studies have discovered modified food genes in the brains of infant mice. This finding has frightening implications. It suggests that genetically modified foods might affect human genetics.

Wind, birds, and insects can carry genetically altered seeds into nearby fields and farther. Pollen from genetically modified plants can cross-pollinate with natural crops. Once GMOs, bacteria, and viruses are dispersed in the environment, it is impossible to control them. The negative effects are irreversible.

Genetically modified organisms cannot be used in organic farming. When you read about the dangers associated with GMOs, you will have even more reasons to eat fresh, organic food.

THE CARE AND FEEDING OF LIVESTOCK

The conventional and organic care and feeding of livestock differ radically. Conventional meat is raised in feedlots. The facilities are like factories that house tens of thousands of animals in deplorable conditions. They are crowded so close together that they can hardly move. Normal behavior is impossible. At some factory farms, animals do not even have space to lie down. Under these conditions, disease can spread quickly. The animals are dosed with antibiotics to keep them from getting sick. Scientists are concerned that the use of antibiotics on feedlots could lead to "superbugs," strains of bacteria that resist antibiotics and can be passed to humans. Organic regulations do not allow medical treatments unless the animal is sick. Organic livestock are not given antibiotics as a preventive measure.

Organic livestock must be fed a diet of organic agricultural products, grass, and grains that have not been sprayed with toxins. Conventionally raised cattle eat soybeans and corn that have been produced with many toxins. Those toxins are stored in the fat cells of cattle. Cattle are meant to eat grass; their digestive system is designed for it. Cattle do not graze at a feedlot. There is no grass. Cattle that are fed grains alone have more deadly E. coli bacteria in their intestines and feces that can contaminate meat during slaughter.

At feedlots, livestock are given growth hormones and other supplements so that they grow faster and can be slaughtered sooner to save the cost of letting the animals develop and grow naturally. When you eat the meat, you absorb the hormones and antibiotics. You already know about the effects of endocrine disrupters on your body. Organically raised livestock is not treated with hormones.

Feedlots hurt the environment. They produce millions of tons of manure that contaminate water supplies. Sometimes conventional farmers collect manure and spray it on the land; this practice can create health problems for people in the area. The *E. coli* present in the manure can contaminate vegetable crops. In organic pastures, where the grass is not treated with synthetic fertilizers or pesticides, manure from the animals is used instead, a practical way to dispose of waste.

> I have had some discoloration on my neck for years and have never been able to get rid of it. It always made me self-conscious. I was told it was the weight that was causing it. Today, I was in the shower scrubbing my neck. All this dead skin just rolled off, lots and lots of it. I was amazed. That discoloration is finally all gone. I'm ecstatic!
>
> T.B.

All this should persuade you that eating organically raised meat and poultry is better for the animals, for you, and for the planet. At this stage, you have cleaned up your act and you are fueling your body with pure and wholesome food. You are ready for healing and restoration with the help of high-density supplements.

Level Three: High-Density Nutritional Supplements

This stage of the 1 Pound a Day Diet Detox differs from all the other cleanses, juice fasts, and so-called detoxes out there. We support your detox with supplements that provide powerful nutrients in small, concentrated amounts. As you eliminate toxins from your body, you will be nourishing every cell with the nutrients of which your body is so often deprived, whether your diet is less than ideal or your body burden is taking its toll. When you consume high-density nutritional supplements, food becomes medicine. The supplements we have incorporated into our program support detoxification, promote weight loss, restore hormonal balance, strengthen the immune system, reduce inflammation, and protect against degenerative disease.

When we talk about supplements, we do not mean synthetic vitamins you buy at the health food, drug, or grocery store. The supplements we use are made from fruits and vegetables that have been concentrated into powdered or liquid form. These supplements are packed with phytonutrients, the components of plants that promote health. We are supposed to eat five to nine servings of fruits and vegetables daily. More than 70 percent of the U.S. population does not meet that requirement. The supplements we recommend will provide you with five or six portions of vegetables and nutrients in one serving. We have made certain that the products we recommend are made from fresh produce that has not been subjected to high temperatures that can damage nutrients. The ingredients are carefully monitored to be sure they are free from contaminants like herbicides and pesticides. If the juice is converted to powder, we verify that the drying process has not damaged the micronutrients.

You will be taking them several times daily to support your detox and nutritional status. Many people continue to take the supplements after finishing the detox, because they provide a boost. We do not mean to suggest that these supplements should replace fresh vegetables and fruits in your diet.

We have our own detox kits available at our website (www.mvdietdetox.com). We also use products by Univera that can be ordered at our website (go to www.mvdietdetox.com and click on Univera.com). We have been using these products and know they are effective. It is also one-stop shopping. We also recommend products and brands that you can find online or at a local vitamin or health food store. We will describe on the following pages the supplements you need to take.

GREEN DRINKS

This high-density supplement packs a wallop. It is primarily made from grasses. Grains like wheat, barley, and rye begin their life cycle as grass. When they are at this stage, they are particularly high in nutrition. That nutrition is much more densely concentrated than it will be when the plants mature. The powder we use at our retreat contains broccoli, greens, kale, spirulina, nutrient-rich algae, and blue-green algae, as well as wheatgrass, an energizer. Wheatgrass is a powerful cleanser and nourishment as well. Some people cannot tolerate drinking it straight until they have detoxified. You see it in shot glasses at juice bars. Warning: a shot of wheatgrass can temporarily turn your teeth and tongue a vivid emerald green.

The grasses and vegetables are harvested at their peak, then dried and converted to powders. Though this is a process, it does not jeopardize the vitamins, minerals, nutrients, phytochemicals, or enzymes. Sometimes sweeter fruits and vegetables—apples, bananas, berries, and carrots—are added for taste. Mixing a scoop or 1½ tablespoons into an eight-ounce glass of water provides you with eight to ten servings of vegetables. You can take the powder with you anywhere in a resealable bag and pour it into your water bottle anytime you are on the run.

Green drinks do so much good for your body. They reduce acidity and lower the risk of certain cancers, diabetes, heart disease, and stroke. The drinks will reduce your appetite, stimulate the loss of body fat, boost your metabolism, improve metal acuity, and protect your memory. You should incorporate green drinks into your normal diet after you have finished detoxing. Look at them as a form of insurance that covers emergencies and protects you from the unpredictable. You will know you are supporting your body with the nutrients it needs to function well.

> **The Best Green Drinks**
>
> The Martha's Vineyard Diet Detox Essential Greens Drink (www.mvdietdetox.com)
>
> Univera MetaGreens (go to www.mvdietdetox and click on Univera)
>
> Dr. Gordon's Organic Best of Greens (www.longevityplus.com)
>
> Allergy Research Group SlimGreens (www.allergyresearchgroup.com)
>
> Garden of Life Perfect Food Super Green Formula (www.gardenoflife.com)

Green grasses contain chlorophyll, a green pigment that absorbs light energy from the sun. Chlorophyll transforms that solar energy into ATP, which transports the energy to cells. When you consume these grasses and other green foods, you are eating sunshine that has been converted to nourishment. Think of the sun's super energy. You get a taste of it every time you eat a green vegetable.

ANTIOXIDANT BERRY DRINKS

Antioxidants counter oxidation, a normal chemical process in the body as the body metabolizes oxygen. When the body is healthy, oxygen metabolism is very efficient. Only 1 to 2 percent of cells will get damaged and turned into free radicals. Oxidative stress occurs when the body's supply of antioxidants is not sufficient to handle and neutralize the free radicals produced by oxidation. Free radicals are unstable molecules that interact aggressively with other molecules and create abnormal cells. External toxins also create free radicals. Drinking alcohol, smoking, and sunbathing can cause an unsafe free radical production. Air pollution, infection, and exposure to toxins throw off the balance in your body, pushing it over the line to oxidative stress. Free radicals can injure cells, damaging DNA and setting the course for disease. They break down tissue and weaken the immune system. When free radicals are out of control, they accelerate aging and contribute to the development of such chronic illnesses as cancer, Alzheimer's disease, Parkinson's disease, cardiovascular disease, cataracts, and macular degeneration.

As you age, your natural defenses against free radicals and oxidative stress become less effective. A high level of antioxidants in your diet can help to prevent age-related diseases. For the detox, you will be taking an antioxidant supplement that provides a high dose of antioxidants, which are naturally found mostly in fruits. They tend to be very colorful. Blueberries, pomegranates, grapes, blackberries, prunes, and raspberries have earned the title "superfoods." You will have berry antioxidants on the detox. They are full of antioxidants that heal inflammation and toxic damage. They reduce joint pain and decrease fluid retention.

Vitamins, minerals, and compounds in food have antioxidant

properties. Vitamins A, C, and E are antioxidants. Beta-carotene, lycopene, and selenium have antioxidant properties as well. We will discuss the whole foods that contain antioxidants in the third part of the book.

You will be taking your antioxidants in liquid form to make absorption easier. Each serving has the nutritional equivalent of six to eight servings of fruit, mostly berries. Choose one containing as many different kinds of berries in it as possible. Go for some new tastes. Try acai berry, wolfberry, goji berry, and noni. This supplement is always popular because it tastes so good.

Recommended Antioxidant Berry Drinks

The Martha's Vineyard Diet Detox Berry Drink (www.mvdietdetox.com)

Univera MetaBerry (go to www.mvdietdetox.com and click on Univera)

Stop Aging Now SuperFruit Elixir Liquid Supplement (www.stopagingnow.com)

Vibrant Health Rainbow Vibrance (www.vibranthealth.us)

If you are shopping for an antioxidant supplement, make certain it has a high ORAC (oxygen radical absorbance capacity) value. ORAC measures the potency of the antioxidants in the drink. The U.S. Food and Drug Administration recommends 7,000 ORAC units daily, the equivalent of five to ten fruits and vegetables. The supplement should not contain added sugar, salt, or preservatives. Look for a drink with a variety of berries.

DIGESTIVE ENZYMES

Enzymes are responsible for every reaction in the body, and play a vital role in the digestive process. They are active proteins that serve as catalysts to bring about change and control biochemical reactions to sustain life. They purify the blood. They keep the colon clean by helping to remove toxic waste. They help to produce neurotransmitters that allow our nervous system to work properly.

The role of digestive enzymes, which are produced in the mouth, stomach, pancreas, and small intestine, is to direct the use of all the nutrients and minerals found in the food we eat. They speed up digestion so that the body can use the nutrients and minerals to function. They break down food into simple sugars, fatty acids, and amino acids and direct the chemical reactions that allow metabolism to happen. They regulate nutrient levels at a normal level.

Enzymes are depleted as you age. According to nutrition experts, you will lose about 13 percent of your enzymes for every decade you live after the age of thirty. Given their importance in maintaining your health, you have to turn around this natural depletion. Your body has a limited ability to produce enzymes. Nature has designed the human body to work with the enzyme content in foods. Enzymes are found only in live, uncooked, unprocessed foods. When food is subjected to a temperature of more than 118°F, the enzymes die. This makes digestion more difficult. All the organs that support the production of natural enzymes—the pancreas, gallbladder, and liver—are forced to work harder to produce extra enzymes. The body is in overdrive to produce them. The food you eat has a direct effect on the depletion of the catalysts that make your body run.

SAD, the standard American diet, consists of many dead foods. Processing foods kills their natural enzymes. When your body no longer produces enough enzymes of its own or there are insufficient enzymes in the food you eat, you experience abdominal pain,

Recommended Enzymes

The enzyme supplement you take should contain protease, amylase, lipase, and cellulose. The products we recommend are:

Univera EnzyDigest
(go to www.mvdietdetox.com and click on Univera)

Twin Lab Super Enzyme Caps
(www.twinlab.com)

Source Naturals Essential Enzymes
(www.sourcenaturals.com)

Pure Encapsulations Digestive Enzymes Ultra (www.pureencapsulations.com)

Vitamin Shoppe Digestive Enzymes
(www.vitaminshoppe.com)

bloating, constipation, gas, and nausea, because what you eat is not being well digested. You can feel weak because nutrients and minerals are not being absorbed well. Other symptoms include headache, extreme fatigue, and decreased energy. Enzymes naturally treat food allergens. When enzymes are depleted, you can develop itching, a rash, or food intolerances.

You have to shift the balance in your everyday diet: Reduce your consumption of cooked and overly processed foods, and eat as much of raw, uncooked vegetables, fruits, and juices as you need to be certain your body has enough enzymes to run smoothly. After you reach age forty, taking enzyme supplements before meals will make your digestion efficient again so that you benefit from the nutrients you consume. While on the detox, you will take enzymes in pill form before having fresh soup.

Recommended Aloe Vera

Garden Greens Inner Cleanse
(www.mvdietdetox.com)

Univera Aloe Gold
(go to www.mvdietdetox.com and click on Univera)

Lily of the Desert Aloe Vera Gel
(www.lilyofthedesert.com)

Swanson Aloe Vera Whole Gel
(www.swansonvitamins.com)

Lakewood Pure Aloe Vera Gel
(www.lakewoodjuices.com)

ALOE VERA

Aloe vera is a succulent with a number of medicinal uses. It has an anti-inflammatory effect. The plant is used as a topical remedy for minor cuts, burns, and skin rashes. Aloe also moisturizes and is used in beauty products for the hair and skin. Keeping a potted aloe vera on the kitchen windowsill is more than just decor.

You will take aloe vera as a nutritional supplement while on the detox. When taken internally, aloe provides antiaging antioxidants, helps to restore pH balance, repairs cellular health, acts as a mild laxative, and improves colon health. Research has shown that aloe is therapeutic with chronic colon conditions like colitis. Aloe vera is hard to find as a concentrated gel, but a gel is preferable to juice.

Recommended Protein Drinks

Univera Meta Fuel (go to www
.mvdietdetox.com and click on Univera)

The Martha's Vineyard Diet Detox Protein
Drink (www.mvdietdetox.com)

Jay Robb Whey Protein or Egg White Protein
(www.jayrobb.com)

NOW Sports Whey Protein Isolate Powder
(www.nowfoods.com)

NOW Egg White Protein Powder
(www.nowfoods.com)

Garden of Life Raw Protein Powder
(www.gardenoflife.com)

PROTEIN DRINKS

If you do not want to lose weight while detoxing, you should have one or two protein drinks a day. We have found that weight loss slows down if you add protein to the detox. As you are doing the nine-day transition from the detox, you will eventually add protein drinks to the regimen. Be certain that the drink has more protein than carbohydrates. Look for a brand made from soy, eggs, and/or whey. Check to see if you are allergic to any of the ingredients.

While detoxing, mix your drink with water or almond, oat, or hemp milk instead of cow's milk. For additional flavor, add natural extracts like vanilla, cinnamon, almond, or banana.

The Best Probiotics

Natren Healthy Trinity (www.natren.com)

Jarrow Formulas Ultra Jarro-Dophilus
(www.jarrow.com)

Health Force Friendly Force, The Ultimate
Probiotic (www.healthforce.com)

PROBIOTICS

Probiotics are good bacteria that help to maintain the natural balance of organisms called microflora in the intestines. The bacteria that live in your gut keep pathogens in check, aid digestion and absorption of nutrients, and boost the immune system.

Probiotics are used to prevent diarrhea, gas, and cramping caused by antibiotics, which kill beneficial bacteria along with the bacteria that cause illness. Taking probiotics like acidophilus can help to replace the good bacteria. Probiotics can lessen the symptoms of colitis, Crohn's disease, and irritable bowel syndrome. Probiotics prevent and treat vaginal yeast infections and urinary tract infections. You will take probiotics while you detox to restore the balance in your digestive tract.

JUMP RIGHT IN OR EASE INTO IT?

Some of you are so fired up that you are ready to start right away. You are ready to go cold turkey and live without coffee, alcohol, meat, bread, and other solid food for almost a month. There is nothing wrong with being ready to dive right in. We are glad that you are eager to start.

Some of you might be a bit apprehensive and want to prepare yourself for the changes you are about to make. If you are in the take-it-slow group, you might need a week to wean yourself from coffee, diet soda, ice cream, and other foods you think might be hard to live without before you begin the detox. You can begin by not eating meat, salt, sugar, and flour, and by increasing the vegetables, fruit, and greens you consume. You might change your mind and decide to begin before the week is up.

Either way you chose to begin, the 1 Pound a Day Diet Detox will work wonders. You will shed pounds, feel energized, and glow with renewed health.

Be honest. Aren't you excited to begin? Following this detox and eating clean has become a way of life for us. Just as we have, you will learn to listen to your body. An unhealthy body gives you signals—headaches, allergies, hypertension, aching joints, and weight gain. If you are like most of us, you manage to ignore those signals like background noise. You feel worse and worse and finally feel so bad that you resolve to do something about it. Sometimes you have to get sick first before you make changes to take care of yourself.

When you detoxify your body as deeply as you are about to do, you will become sensitized. You will be lighter in weight and in

> At church this past Sunday, I got five compliments from people telling me I was literally "glowing"—I was so excited! People thought I was pregnant because I had a glow!
>
> J.V.

spirit. You will like what you see in the mirror and so will your family and friends. You will be feeling upbeat and full of life. Those nagging symptoms and physical problems will have vanished.

You will want to stay that way. You will notice when your body is veering toward toxic overload. You will feel subtle shifts in your overall well-being. In *1 Pound a Day*, you have a practical plan to return to super health anytime you feel the need. That is one of the reasons we suggest you do an annual detox. Make it a regular event each year. Pick a start date and put it on your calendar when a new year begins. Some detoxers like to pull themselves together after the excesses of the holidays, to start the year off right. Others like to come out of winter with a detox in the early spring. Whatever suits you is perfect. Staying healthy is a continuing process, and toxins do not take a break. You owe it to yourself to keep your body in top working condition. You deserve to look and feel fabulous all the time.

> I injured my right knee playing tennis in 2009 and for some reason it wouldn't heal. After my detox, my right knee is so much better, and I can move laterally on the tennis court again. I've never felt better—never—than when I did the detox.
>
> K.E.

Detox Success Story

NOTHING WILL MAKE ME GAIN WEIGHT THIS TIME

I am a Brazilian living in Atlanta, Georgia. I did the diet detox in 2008 and 2012. One day, I stepped on the scale and I saw 200 pounds. I thought, "No way. I am not letting this happen to me." So I started my search for a healthy diet. That's when I found your first book, *21 Pounds in 21 Days*, online. I read the book cover to cover, highlighting what was most important to me. I ordered my supplements and bought everything else I needed. I remember my supplements arrived on a Tuesday. I told my Mom I would start on a Monday. She replied, "Why? You have everything. Just start tomorrow." So I did.

I was so excited by what I was doing that I didn't have the healing crisis described in the book. The first week passed quickly. When I looked down at the scale and saw 192 pounds, I couldn't believe it. That got me extra motivated. With more energy to keep going, I was feeling relieved and happy. I told my family, "I can do it. I will do it."

I measured my body—two to three inches gone every week. And the teeth—oh, wow—I just loved my white teeth and smooth smile. Since you are not chewing anything, you get that healthy and glowing appearance. All of a sudden, I was done. I lost twenty-four pounds in twenty-one days and continued to drop another five pounds during maintenance.

I am so glad I did the detox. It really changed me. I am very calm now and have more energy. I think clearly. When I started to eat again, I tried to chew the food slowly. I counted how many pounds I had to lose and chewed my food that many times.

The first time I did the detox in 2008, I started at 216 pounds and went down to 148 pounds in a year. After a horrible breakup, I started to gain weight again. This time, when I saw 200 pounds on the scale, I promised myself I would not go back to this weight again. I promised myself that I would not let anyone or anything make me gain a pound. From my 200 pounds, I went down to 176 pounds. During transition I lost another five pounds. My goal is 140 pounds. I did it once. I can do it again.

Larissa Oliviera

PART 2

THE
1 POUND A DAY
DIET DETOX

CHAPTER 4

⌒

THE GAME PLAN

You are about to take positive steps to get control of your weight, to lift the level of your health, and to rid yourself of the nagging symptoms of toxic overload that have become part of your life. When people come to the Martha's Vineyard Holistic Retreat to detox, we talk about why they want to do the program and what they want to achieve. You should consider the same things at home. Before you begin the program, you should set some goals for yourself. You should assess how you feel and look right now, your current condition. You should consider:

- What has made you decide to detox?
- Do you dread not chewing for a month?
- What foods will you miss the most?
- Could your lifestyle be healthier?
- Do you want to lose weight? If so, how much?
- Have you gained weight around the middle?
- Do you want to get your energy back?
- Do you want to sleep better?
- Do you look tired?
- Are your skin and hair dull?
- Do you have any routine and recurrent health problems, like headaches, aching joints, allergies, indigestion?

- Do you just feel off?
- Do you worry that you are going to get sick?
- Do any diseases run in your family that you want to try to avoid?
- Do you have any chronic diseases like asthma, arthritis, diabetes, high blood pressure, high cholesterol, heart disease, cancer?
- Do you want to recapture the way you used to look and feel?

You get the idea. Just jot down what has been bothering you that you want to change. Listing and visualizing what you want to change can help the process.

It is a good idea to record your progress in an informal journal. Many detoxers take photos of themselves that they post on the refrigerator and tape onto the inside cover of their journal. There is nothing like before-and-after pictures to show you what you have achieved. Seeing the difference will make it easy to commit to long-term change. You can take before-and-after videos of yourself and post them on YouTube. You could inspire other detoxers if you posted your before-and-after shots on any of our social media links, including Twitter, Facebook, Pheed, and YouTube, which is our website www.mvdietdetox .com. Just click on the icon of your choice and share your pho-

I just finished the detox and lost thirty pounds in twenty-one days. I am eating healthy now and working out. I am going to wait about four weeks as my girlfriend wants to do it also. All I can say is WOW, this really works. The thing is, I am doing it for myself first. It takes a lot of dedication to do this detox and stay away from food.

Now that I am eating again, it's just unbelievable how much I used to actually eat. Take before pictures in swimming trunks and post it on your fridge for incentive. I have an after picture, and all I can say is Wow again. You can do this. I did.

S.H.

tos and experiences. You will find a community who will help you to celebrate how great you look and feel.

When you keep a daily journal, you will have a clear idea of how you are progressing toward those goals. Record your weight each morning. Take your measurements the day you start the detox. Record your measurements, especially your waist, on the same day each week. The pounds and inches will melt away. As you experience remarkable changes during your month of detox, you will be motivated to stay with it.

Each day, you should record how you are feeling physically and emotionally, good and bad. Make note if you feel yourself wanting to cheat. Sometimes writing it down will stop the impulse. Keeping track of the improvements is encouraging. When you have finished the detox and are following Dr. Roni's Healthy Eating Plan, you can look back to remind yourself of where you started. You definitely will not want to go back there.

DETOX FUNDAMENTALS

The 1 Pound a Day Diet Detox is built on three simple principles:

1. Consuming maximum nutrition in small doses
2. Nourishing your body every two hours
3. Consuming all nutrients in liquid form

On the detox, you will be consuming the equivalent of at least twenty-two servings of fruits and vegetables in the form of soups, fresh juices, and supplements. That is well above the USDA recommendation of five to nine servings a day.

The detox is designed to avoid starving your body, which is what most diets do, leading to weight-loss resistance. Instead, you will be providing your cells with a steady supply of dense nutrients that keep your blood sugar even and turn your body into a fat-burning machine. As much as you might doubt it now, you will not be hungry once the cleanse kicks in after two to three days. Your body is getting what it has been starved for.

By not eating solid foods, you allow your digestive system to rest. If your intestines are not involved in processing the solid food you normally eat, the cleanse will be deeper. At the same time, the energy normally expended to metabolize food can be directed to repairing cell damage and rebuilding.

Drinking plenty of water is essential to flush out the toxins that are released. If you do not, the toxins will be recirculated and stored again in your fat cells. Using distilled water during the detox is very important. Tap water is often treated with fluoride and contains hard minerals that can lead to hardening of the arteries. Even bottled spring water contains traces of calcium, sodium, potassium, fluoride, magnesium, bicarbonate, nitrate, chloride, copper, sulfate, arsenic, and lead. The process of distillation removes many impurities from water. The water is boiled and the steam is condensed into a clean container. While you are purifying your body, it does not make sense to use anything but pure distilled water.

You will use distilled water during the detox to mix your supplements, to make your teas, broths, and soups, and to drink when you are thirsty. You will go through many gallon jugs of distilled water in the next thirty days. When you are out and about and distilled water is not available, you can resort to bottled water. You should try to plan ahead and carry a water bottle filled with distilled water. Even with the best intentions, we all slip up sometimes, but don't make a habit of it. Remember: you will achieve the best results by following the thirty-day program as closely as you can.

You will not want to be too far from a bathroom, particularly in the early days of the detox. Your body will be eliminating toxins rapidly along with all the fluids you consume.

THE DAILY PLAN

At this point, you have learned so much about the 1 Pound a Day Diet Detox that you probably want to see what a day on the detox actually looks like. You can copy the schedule that follows and post it on your refrigerator, put a copy in your journal, and carry one with you in a purse or briefcase, or folded up in a back pocket. James suggests setting the alarm on your phone to ring every two hours to remind you it is time to nourish your body. Start the boxed schedule that follows no later than an hour after you wake up.

Some of our detoxers tell us that they love having so few choices. They enjoy not having to think about food. As the detox goes on, you will find yourself getting more creative about juicing combinations and using herbs and spices in the soup and broth for flavor. The next two chapters will give you some ideas and some excellent recipes.

You can drink water, tea, and vegetable broth interchangeably anytime you want during the day. We have scheduled them to make certain you drink enough fluids to support your cleanse. At the retreat, we have a slow cooker going all day to make broth. We will discuss this in detail in Chapter 7. The more you drink, the easier it will be for you to lose weight.

HOW 1 POUND A DAY WORKS

This detox is designed to cleanse and to heal. Your body will release toxins that have been stored in your organs and fat cells into your bloodstream, where they will travel to the organs of elimination and be processed out of your body. The large quantity of vegetables that you will be consuming contains nutrients that cleanse your cells. Green vegetables are particularly cleansing. Dark green vegetables get their color from chlorophyll, a chemical compound that collects light and uses the light to create plant energy. Chlorophyll and the leafy vegetables in which it's found are superfoods with powerful benefits.

THE 1 POUND A DAY DIET DETOX

8:00 a.m.
> Probiotic
> High-density antioxidant berry drink
> 8 ounces of distilled water
> Hot herbal tea (lemon or stevia optional)

10:00 a.m.
> High-density green drink mixed in 8 ounces of distilled water
> 8 ounces of distilled water or "free soup" or vegetable broth or
>   herbal tea*

12:00 noon
> Fresh vegetable juice or another high-density green drink
> 8 ounces of distilled water or vegetable broth or herbal tea*

2:00 p.m.
> High-density green drink mixed in 8 ounces of distilled water
> 8 ounces of distilled water or vegetable broth or herbal tea*

4:00 p.m.
> High-density antioxidant berry drink
> 8 ounces of distilled water or vegetable broth or herbal tea*

6:00 p.m.
> 1 enzyme capsule with sip of distilled water
> Homemade soup
> Broth from soup
> Herbal tea

8:00 p.m.
> 8 ounces of distilled water or vegetable broth or herbal tea*

Bedtime
> Aloe vera or herbal cleanse with 4 ounces of distilled water

*On the detox, you can substitute homemade vegetable broth for distilled water or light herbal tea.

Everyone has different fluid requirements. If you are urinating a light yellow–tinged color about every two hours, you have met your fluid requirements. You may also drink your fluids on the odd hours.

Chlorophyll is the plant equivalent of hemoglobin in red blood cells. Hemoglobin carries oxygen to the cells. With a similar composition, chlorophyll acts the same way in your body. With more oxygen transported to your cells, energy is produced and toxins are released as metabolism occurs.

Chlorophyll is a potent antioxidant. In that capacity, chlorophyll reduces inflammation and free radicals. That action has a beneficial effect on arthritis and other inflammatory diseases. Your immune cells are more effective when the free radical count is lowered. Chlorophyll helps your body to destroy and eliminate germs and to prevent new germ growth.

The compound is believed to reduce the risk of certain forms of cancer by binding to carcinogens your body has a difficult time absorbing. Your body is able to eliminate the new complex formed by the chlorophyll. Employing a similar chemical interaction, chlorophyll is able to bind with highly toxic heavy metals like mercury and remove those metals from your body.

In addition to being a deodorizer, chlorophyll aids in digestion and reduces constipation. As you can see, chlorophyll is good for you in every way. While you are detoxing, you will feel the benefits almost immediately. Drinking green juices and consuming dark leafy greens for the rest of your life is a habit you will be happy to form, because the effects are extraordinary.

The food-based, nutritionally dense supplements that you will be taking, plus the juice and soup during the detox, far exceed your daily nutritional needs. Your body will not signal your brain for nutrition. Instead, your body can focus on expelling harmful chemicals and the fat that houses so many of them.

REBUILDING, RESTORING, HEALING

The 1 Pound a Day Diet Detox goes beyond ridding your body of damaging toxins. The program supports your body in reversing the damage that has been done and in regenerating new, healthy cells. Nourishing yourself with liquids only—no chewing allowed for the first twenty-one days—saves energy. When you eat a normal meal, your body has to work hard to digest it and transport the nutrients to the cells. When all your food is in liquid form, the process of breaking down the food is easier. Supplying nourishment to the cells is more efficient. More energy is produced and less is expended in the process.

We do not often think about how much energy is spent digesting what we eat. We are accustomed to a slump after a meal or sweet snack but do not make the connection. The fact is that digesting food demands more energy than any other process in the body. The liquid diet of the detox changes all that. You will be amazed by how much excess energy you suddenly have. Many detoxers describe it as a feeling of total rejuvenation.

The detox gives the healing capacity of your body a boost. The energy that had been used to digest food is available to repair toxic damage while you are on the program. At the same time, you are consuming more nutrients than you need for your body to function well. The excess of easily accessible nutrients is put to good use. Once the toxins begin to be eliminated, the surplus of nutrients and the increased available energy are directed to cells, tissues, and organs that have been damaged to help them repair and recover.

> Before the detox my eyes were really bad. I wear glasses, but do not like to wear them, so my eyes have gotten worse. The last time I had my exam I needed a stronger prescription. The other day I was looking for something in my car and found my prescription for my glasses. I realized I had not had any issues with my eyes since I started the detox. This is Day 14, and I feel amazing. I can see things I could not see before. No squinting, no headaches—awesome!
>
> Beth Clark

The detox reverses the constant tearing-down action of toxins. Your body will have all it needs to build new, healthy cells. This renewed power will be immediately noticeable in the way your skin looks. Your skin is constantly exposed to toxins from the air, from water, from grooming products, from the sun. High toxic levels are visible on your face. A high body burden ages your skin. When your body is in healing mode, the quality of your skin will change. Very early in the detox process, you will see signs that your skin is revitalized. You will look refreshed. Detoxers say that years are removed from their faces. Age spots fade, wrinkles disappear, and the glow returns. Many who had considered cosmetic surgery no longer think they need it. If that level of transformation is happening on the surface, imagine what is going on inside your body. Every organ, and every cell, is undergoing major restoration. Your body has served you well. You are giving it the ultimate payback by doing the 1 Pound a Day Diet Detox.

The next chapter will give you advice on how to get organized for the detox, so that you have everything in place when you begin.

Detox Success Story
NO MORE VENTI LATTES

I'm starting my fifth detox today, my second full detox. When I started my first detox two years ago, I was desperate. A dietitian by trade, I couldn't understand why I had been so sick for approximately ten years with hives, headaches, blisters, sinus infections—the list goes on—and taking nine meds each day . . .

Desperate, I agreed to try the Martha's Vineyard Diet Detox, which was recommended by a friend . . . After all, I was a dietitian. After the first week of detox, all my hives and blisters were healing. The second week was more challenging, but I struggled through because my hives were now gone. By the end of week three, I had so much energy. This was a crazy concept for me, because I was used to four venti lattes daily for energy. Now I was glowing and bouncing off walls.

. . . I never went back to either wheat or dairy after that detox. I was able to drop all meds except my birth control. Turns out I'm not depressed and my health problems were due to my diet . . .

Even though I work in the health care field, I now know that allopathic medicine has its place . . . The book has truly saved my life, both mentally and physically.

B.G.

CHAPTER 5

THE SETUP

Starting a detox is like cooking from a recipe. You line up all the ingredients and read the directions before you begin. Nothing is more frustrating than discovering as you are cooking that the key ingredient you thought you had in the cupboard is not there, or you should have soaked the beans overnight, or one of the steps of the recipe requires ninety minutes of cooking time that you had not noticed. You need to know what you have to do before you start to cook. If you are prepared before you begin the program, you will fly through the month without stress. You have decided to do something good for yourself. You want the experience to be as rewarding as possible. Just a little bit of planning will make your detox month effortless. As we said earlier, doing the detox should not be a part-time job. This chapter will give you some tried-and-true tips for getting ready.

RUN IT BY YOUR DOCTOR

Before you start any detox or diet, you should consult with your doctor about your plans. If you have a chronic illness, it is even more important for you to do so. We have heard from many de-toxers that their doctors initially had a knee-jerk reaction. They thought the detox was extreme and unnecessary, because they had learned that the body detoxes itself. You have to put this response in perspective. For the most part, medical doctors have not been educated on the subjects of nutrition, weight loss, and detoxification. In light of the obesity epidemic, that is beginning to change. Medical schools have only recently included nutrition and weight loss in the curriculum.

If your doctor dismisses the detox, explain the principles. You will be forming new eating habits and will be dropping processed and fast food from your diet. You will be taking high-density anti-oxidants and other supplements and drinking fresh vegetable juice for a month. You will be significantly increasing your consumption of vegetables, which are packed with vitamins and minerals. There is nothing unhealthy about any of this.

PICK A DATE TO BEGIN

Look at your calendar and find a thirty-day period without too many social demands. If you do this far enough in advance, you can keep your calendar open by scheduling only social events and business travel that are unavoidable. Being at a fine restaurant, at a holiday meal, or at a dinner party can be very challenging when you are detoxing. We will give you tips later about how to handle the temptations of a number of social situations.

We recommend that first-time detoxers begin the detox on a Tuesday. Between the third and seventh day, most people experience what we call a "healing crisis," which we cover in detail in Chapter 8. You might feel off at that point in the program, as toxins are released from storage and enter your bloodstream and organs. Symptoms range from headaches to fatigue to irritability and being down in the dumps. The intensity of your healing crisis often depends on the degree of your toxicity. By starting on a Tuesday, you will not have your busy week disrupted by being under the weather. Your healing crisis is likely to occur during the weekend, when there are fewer demands on your time and energy. You can slow down and let your body deal with eliminating all the toxins that are being released. You will begin the next week with a noticeable change in your stamina and spirit and will sail through the remainder of the detox in great form.

GET YOUR SUPPLEMENTS FIRST

Whether your supplements and green drink powder are being mail-ordered or you are buying them locally, you should leave enough time for shipment or to find the recommended brands, two weeks before you start the detox. You will need

- Antioxidant berry drink (products listed on page 51)
- Green drink powder (products listed on page 49)
- Aloe vera (products listed on page 53)
- Protein drinks (products listed on page 54)
- Enzymes (products listed on page 52)
- Probiotics (products listed on page 54)
- Omega-3 pills or flaxseed oil (you will add fatty acids on Day 25, the fourth day of your transition)
- Several gallons of distilled water (figure at least 64 ounces or a half-gallon a day)

DETOX EQUIPMENT

You will need two small appliances; a third is optional.

- Juicer
- Blender or food processor
- Slow cooker (optional)

Since you are going to be having fresh juice for lunch during your detox, you will need a juicer to ensure that your juice is organic and fresh. Making your own juice is less expensive than buying it at a health food store or a juice bar. After you have completed the detox, juicing is part of Dr. Roni's Healthy Eating Plan, so the investment is long term.

To puree vegetables for your evening soup, you will need a blender or food processor.

At the retreat, we keep broth in a slow cooker to make what we call "free soup" available all day. Detoxers can have a cup of the broth whenever they want. You can use a slow cooker or accomplish the same thing with a pot with a cover that sits on a back burner to keep warm. Just make sure to add fresh distilled water now and then.

You probably do not already own a juicer, so this is what to look for.

Buying a Juicer

When we talk about a juicer, we do not mean a citrus juicer, in which you press halves of fruit on a reamer. What you need to make fresh vegetable juice is a juice extractor. There are three types of juicers on the market:

Centrifugal juicers use a quickly spinning disk that cuts fruit or vegetables into very small pieces that are spun to separate the juice from the pulp. The juice flows through a strainer and into a container. Centrifugal juicers are reasonably priced. They tend to be noisy. The fast-moving blades juice quickly, but the fast shredding is said to oxidize the juice, depleting some nutrients. The heat generated can destroy enzymes. It is important to drink juices produced this way immediately.

Masticating or cold press juicers have a single slowly rotating presser that crushes produce and squeezes out the juice. This type of juicer is excellent for juicing leafy greens. Masticating juicers have the capacity to make nut pastes from soaked nuts and seeds, and fruit sorbets, which makes them useful for Dr. Roni's Healthy Eating Plan. They operate more slowly than centrifugal juicers, and that allows the juice to retain more nutrients. Juicers of this type will produce more juice from fruits and vegetables than a centrifugal juicer. They operate more quietly than centrifugal juicers.

- Cold press juicers come in upright (vertical) and horizontal models. Horizontal juicers take up more counter space than other juicers. The horizontal juicer is the easiest to clean because of its small screen. The upright juicer has a larger screen to clean.
- Masticating juicers are made with a single gear or twin gears.

Triturating juicers, or twin-gear juicers, produce the most nutrient-dense juices. The slow-speed juicers retain the maximum amount of nutrients in the juices because they prevent the produce from being oxidized. The twin-gear juicer is expensive and harder to clean. For your purposes, a centrifugal or single-gear masticating juicer will be all you need.

There are certain features you should look for in a juicer that will make juicing easier.

- A large chute or feeder tube saves time because you do not have to cut up vegetables and fruit. Three inches is ideal.
- Buy the juicer with the most powerful motor you can get in your price range. Insufficient power will cause your motor to slow when you are juicing hard vegetables. You should not buy a juicer with less power than 450 watts.
- A multispeed juicer can save wear and tear on the motor and can handle a greater variety of fruits and vegetables.

- Look for a juicer that is easy to clean, with dishwasher-safe parts. Juicing can be messy. If you can afford it, a juicer with stainless steel parts will not discolor and will last longer.
- Look at the specs to see what percentage of juice versus pulp and waste the juicer yields. Juices that eject the pulp outside the machine yield less juice than juicers that keep the pulp in the basket.
- Check the warranty. A good juicer is guaranteed for five to ten years. Inexpensive juicers are warrantied for ninety days to a year. The cutting blade of an inexpensive juicer can wear out after two to four months of use. There is also a high incidence of motor burnout in less expensive juicers.
- Make sure you can replace parts easily. A juicer is an investment, an appliance you will be using to stay healthy. You want a juicer with longevity.

Spend the time to do some comparative shopping online to get the best price for your juicer. There are often good sales. Another option is to see what is available on eBay. You can pick up a new, barely used, or refurbished juicer at a significant saving. If you make the effort to find a good deal, you will be able to buy a higher-quality juicer without blowing your budget.

Other Supplies That Will Make the Detox a Breeze

With the help of other detoxers, we have developed some practical tips that will help you tackle the detox. A few items will help you organize your vegetables for the day and make your detox portable.

- BPA-free, stainless-steel, or glass food storage containers
- A thermos to carry soup or broth with you
- Stainless-steel or BPA-free plastic water bottles

Juicers to Consider

There are so many juicers available that sorting through them all can be a confusing chore. We have put together a list of the highest-rated and most recommended juicers.

CENTRIFUGAL JUICERS

Breville Juice Fountain Elite 800JEXL is the top of the line. Breville makes a variety of state-of-the-art juicers at a range of price points. They have a big chute and eject pulp.

Omega 1000, 4000, and 9000 are powerful juicers that keep shredded veggies in the basket for more juice. Drawback: a small chute.

Omega Mega Mouth 330 Juicer has a pulp ejector and a big feeder.

Omega 02 Juicer has a pulp ejector.

Acme 5001 and 6001 are comparable to the Omega juicers. This company has been making durable juicers for decades.

Hamilton Beach offers a selection of low-priced juice extractors in the HealthSmart and Big Mouth lines. The Hamilton Beach Big Mouth Pro 67650 has great reviews.

Jack LaLanne PowerJuicers are sold in several models. They have the benefit of a big chute. The shredded vegetables are ejected into a basket, making for easy cleanup. The juicers are well-priced.

Juiceman products are available in several models. They do not eject the pulp. These juicers are relatively inexpensive.

MASTICATING OR COLD PRESS JUICERS

<u>Single Gear</u>

Omega HD VRT350 Juicer (vertical)

Omega 8004/8006 (horizontal)

Hurom HU-100 (upright)

Samson 6 in 1 Wheatgrass Juicer

Tribest Solo Star II Multipurpose Juicer

Lexen Electric Healthy Juicer

Twin Gear

Green Power KPE-1304

Green Power Gold GP-E1503

Green Star Tribest GS-3000

Green Star Elite GSE-5000

Super Angel 5500

On the detox and in the future, you should replace plastic bags and food storage containers with glass, stainless steel, or BPA-free plastic. According to their websites, Tupperware and Rubbermaid make BPA-free storage containers. Pyrex storage containers are a very good choice. You do not have to change everything at once, but do the best you can gradually.

Everyone is always on the go. The demands of your life do not stop when you detox. Make it easy on yourself by being ready to take the detox on the road. You can take broth or soup with you in a thermos in the car or at the office. If you have two water bottles filled with distilled water, you can make the antioxidant berry or green drink at the office or when you are not at home during your detox. You do not have to be under house arrest to detox successfully.

OUT WITH THE PROCESSED FOOD

Now is the time to go through your kitchen cabinets and pantry with a toxin detector. Cookies, crackers, chips, dips, cake mixes, white bread and rolls, lunch meats, hot dogs, frozen and canned food, salad dressings, marinades, sauces, soups, sweet breakfast cereals, hard candy, chocolate, and junk foods all have to go. You know the harmful additives and preservatives to look for. You can refer to the list in Chapter 3.

If you have a family, this is more of a challenge. It is almost impossible to make a clean sweep. The other family members will continue to eat their normal diets as you detox. What you have to do is to get rid of the "treats" that will most tempt you, your special stash of goodies. When you start making life changes on Dr. Roni's Healthy Eating Plan, you can gradually shape your family's eating habits by serving wholesome, fresh food. You will be a stellar example of the benefits of eating well. To play on that classic line from *When Harry Met Sally*, it is not uncommon for family members and friends to say, "I'll have what she's having!"

THE SHOPPING LIST

The day before you begin the detox, stock up on the foods that you will be eating. When you buy vegetables, find the freshest produce available. Vegetables can lose up to 45 percent of their nutritional value between the time they are picked and when they land in the produce section of the grocery store. This is one of the reasons it makes sense to buy locally grown vegetables.

I went shopping for everything I needed for twenty-one days and estimated how much distilled water and herbal tea I needed. I purchased two water bottles with measurements for my drinks. I packed the powder mixes in snack bags and labeled them for the week. I took at least four gallons of water to keep at work and two at my business. I didn't drink faucet water. Even in my car trunk I had my distilled water, just in case.

Petrina Devon Young

⌢

Fruits and vegetables will lose nutrients even in your refrigerator. We suggest that you buy enough produce to last three days. If you can shop only once a week, make sure to use the less-hardy vegetables first. Broccoli and celery will hold up longer than chard or spinach. The rule of thumb is never to let your food wilt. If you have to store food before eating it, make sure to refrigerate it immediately. One study showed that kale lost 89 percent of its vitamin C when left at 70°F for two days after picking, compared to 5 percent when stored at a cold temperature for the same period of time. Some vegetables do better left at room temperature, including onions, garlic, and tomatoes. These fruits and vegetables are shocked by the cold and lose nutrients.

Nutrient Loss from Field to Plate

Fruits and vegetables begin to lose nutrients the moment they are picked. These statistics are eye-opening.

Food	Days from Field to Plate	Typical Nutrient Loss
Carrots	9–10	10%
Garden peas	8–10	15%
Broccoli and cauliflower	6–16	25%
Green beans	11–15	45%

That is why we recommend buying local produce that is in season and eating fresh vegetables soon after purchase. When fruits and vegetables are picked at the peak of harvesttime and travel a shorter distance, the produce is fresher, juicier, and more flavorful. Local and seasonal produce is ripened longer on the plant, so it has higher levels of nutrients and flavor than produce that is picked early and ripened artificially. Aside from being more delicious and nutrient-rich, produce bought from farmers' markets will save you money, because you eliminate the middleman. Even better, you support local farmers.

For convenience, you might want to chop up your ingredients and store them in airtight containers. We do not recommend storing cut-up produce for more than three days while you are detoxing, because you are going for maximum nutrition. When any part of a vegetable except its skin is exposed to air, the vegetable loses nutrients rapidly, particularly the antioxidant vitamins C and E. And remember, unless you have bought local produce, your raw food has already spent some time traveling to your grocery store.

On Dr. Roni's Healthy Eating Plan, you should use freshly cut fruits within two or three days and vegetables within four or five days. If at all possible, you should wait to cut up your vegetables each time you juice or make a soup or broth during your detox. It really does not involve that much chopping—especially if you have a juicer with a large feed tube.

The following are the groceries you will need for your detox.

Herbal Teas

You can drink as much herbal tea as you would like during your detox. The only restriction is that your tea should be caffeine-free, although green tea is allowed. Even though green tea contains a small amount of caffeine, it is a good source of antioxidants. Treat yourself to a variety of herbal teas. Feel free to use fresh lemon or stevia as a sweetener. You can sweeten your tea with stevia, extracted from the stevia plant, as a healthy sugar substitute. It comes in liquid and powdered form. Stevia has no calories and is up to thirty or more times sweeter than sugar, so use it sparingly. Get rid of all those pink, yellow, and blue packets. Those sugar substitutes are bad for your body (look back to page 34). For extra flavor try fresh mint, which is especially delicious in iced tea.

Herbal teas have healing properties. This recipe for one of Dr. Roni's homemade herbal teas is great for circulation and metabolism. It is anti-inflammatory and antibacterial. This tea warms the body, tastes great, and fills your kitchen with a homey aroma.

DR. RONI'S CLOVE NUTMEG TEA

2 servings

2 cups distilled water
1 whole clove
2 whole cardamom pods
1 cinnamon stick
¼ teaspoon ground nutmeg, or to taste
Pea-size piece fresh ginger
⅛ teaspoon organic vanilla extract
Stevia

1. In a saucepan, preferably stainless-steel or glass, combine the water, clove, cardamom, cinnamon, nutmeg, and ginger. Simmer gently for 20 minutes.

2. Strain through a fine-mesh sieve into two cups. Add the vanilla and stevia to taste.

You may add your favorite herbal tea bag for extra strength in the last 5 minutes of simmering.

If you are not detoxing, you can use filtered water and add almond milk at the end to make the tea creamy.

Herbs, Spices, and Flavorings

Herbs and spices will add variety to your soups and broths, and fresh herbs add a kick when you juice them for your green drink. You should have these in your spice rack and refrigerator.

Basil*
Bay leaf
Caraway
Cardamom
Cayenne pepper
Cilantro (sometimes known as fresh coriander)*
Cinnamon
Cloves
Cumin
Curry powder
Dill*
Fennel seeds
Flavored stevia
Garlic*
Mint*
Mustard
Oregano*
Rosemary*

Saffron
Sage*
Stevia
Thyme*
Turmeric
No-salt vegetable seasoning
Vanilla (organic extract)

*These are best used fresh for juicing.

In addition, Bragg Liquid Aminos seasoning is a great source of protein.

You do not have to be a gourmet chef to use a wide variety of herbs and spices in your cooking. We encourage you to experiment with them during your detox. Spicing up your juices, soups, broths, and teas will add a new dimension to the pure foods you are consuming. The flavor and aroma of the foods will be richer and more satisfying. You will get so good at using herbs and spices that you will cook chef-worthy dishes when you are on Dr. Roni's Healthy Eating Plan. To encourage you, in the third part of the book we include suggestions on how to cook with herbs and spices and which combinations work well. Your family will certainly appreciate your new cooking savvy. Who knows? You might be ready for the Food Network.

Spices and herbs have remarkable healing properties. They not only make your food taste better but will help your body restore itself. Herbs and spices are natural medicines that prevent and reverse disease. What follows is an overview of the top twenty healing herbs and spices and their health benefits. You can pick and choose according to your health concerns as well as your taste. If you have a condition you want to be rid of or to avoid developing, consider these herbs and spices as powerful medicine.

TWENTY HERBS, SPICES, AND AROMATICS THAT BOOST HEALING

Basil

Basil is rich in antioxidants. The herb is antimicrobial, fighting the germs than can cause colds. It contains a compound called eugenol, which has a calming effect shown to ease muscle spasms. This herb helps to relieve gas and soothe stomach upsets.

Cayenne Pepper

Capsaicin, an oily compound, is responsible for the burning sensation in your mouth when you eat food spiced with cayenne (red) pepper. Capsaicin is the active ingredient in many creams, ointments, and patches for arthritis and muscle pain. It is also used for treating shingles and diabetes-related nerve pain.

As a cold remedy, cayenne relieves congestion by shrinking blood vessels in your nose and throat. It boosts your metabolism, speeding up your calorie burning for a couple of hours after you eat. Cayenne acts as an antioxidant and fights inflammation. Studies have found that it has some cancer-fighting properties and antidiabetes effects. So spice it up. Cayenne adds heat with a healthy punch.

Cilantro (Coriander)

Cilantro is a wonder herb with powerful phytonutrients. It aids digestion, combats allergies, and lowers cholesterol. But that is not all. Cilantro works to reduce inflammation and fight diabetes.

Cinnamon

Cinnamon bark contains cinnamaldehyde, an antibacterial chemical that kills *E. coli*, salmonella, and *Staphylococcus aureus*. Research shows that cinnamon is able to stop the growth of the Asian flu virus. It improves insulin function and lowers blood sugar. By keeping your blood sugar under control, cinnamon helps to prevent diabetes. As little as a half-teaspoon a day may help improve cellular sugar intake and insulin use.

Cinnamon is rich in antioxidants called polyphenols, which fight inflammation. As little as ¼ to ½ teaspoon a day can reduce triglyceride and total cholesterol levels. The active ingredients are known to have a tranquilizing effect that can help to reduce anxiety and stress.

Cloves

Cloves relieve arthritis pain. They contain a phytochemical that interferes with a protein that has been linked to arthritis and other inflammatory diseases. Cloves have been used for centuries to reduce tooth pain. Cloves also contain eugenol.

Cumin

Cumin fights the development and spread of cancer. This spice inhibits the enzymes that help cancer cells invade healthy tissue. It also prevents tumors from developing new blood vessels to help them grow. Cumin has antioxidant properties as well.

Dill

Dill has a soothing affect. It has been used to treat heartburn, colic, and gas for thousands of years.

Fennel Seeds

Fennel seeds have many health-benefiting nutrients, compounds, antioxidants, minerals, and vitamins, most notably high amounts of flavonoid antioxidants. These antioxidants help to protect your body from cancers, infections, heart disease, high cholesterol, stroke, aging, and other degenerative diseases. Fennel seeds are anti-inflammatory, facilitate digestion, and prevent and treat flatulence. Fennel seeds can not only help prevent and treat constipation, but can also act as a laxative with their high fiber content. The oils in fennel have antiacidic properties. Studies have also shown that fennel may inhibit the formation of certain tumors caused by cancer-causing chemicals.

Garlic

Allicin, a sulfur compound, is responsible for most of garlic's broad range of medicinal benefits. When eaten daily, garlic can help to lower the risk of heart disease by as much as 76 percent. It reduces cholesterol levels as well as blood pressure, prevents blood clots by thinning the blood, and acts as an antioxidant. Studies suggest that garlic may prevent the onset of cancer, particularly stomach and colorectal cancers. The sulfur compounds are believed to flush out cancer-causing agents before they can damage DNA, and to cause existing cancer cells to self-destruct. Garlic is strongly antibacterial and antifungal, combating bacteria and viruses that cause earaches, colds, flu, and yeast infections. It can even repel ticks.

Ginger

Ginger is a gnarled rhizome that has been used as a digestive aid in Asian and Indian medicine for centuries. It works in the digestive tract to boost digestive juices, neutralize acids, and reduce intestinal contractions. It is an effective nausea remedy; studies have shown that ginger works just as well as Dramamine to prevent or stop nausea. It combats inflammation and lowers cholesterol.

Mint

Herbalists use mint as a stomach tonic to treat nausea and vomiting, calm stomach muscle spasms, promote digestion, and relieve flatulence. Menthol, the aromatic oil in peppermint, fights bacteria and viruses and opens the airways. Menthol reduces headache pain by interfering with the sensation from pain receptors. There is evidence that peppermint can kill microorganisms and increase mental alertness.

Mustard

Mustard is a plant from the cabbage family. Compounds in mustard seeds may inhibit the growth of cancer cells. It has the heat to break up congestion just as cayenne pepper does; this is why mustard was used in chest plasters. It depletes nerve cells of a chemical that transmits pain signals to the brain when used externally. Mustard stimulates appetite by increasing saliva and digestive juices. Consuming more than a teaspoon of mustard seeds can have a strong laxative effect.

Nutmeg

Like basil and cloves, nutmeg contains eugenol, a compound that benefits the heart. Nutmeg is the seed of an evergreen tree. The covering of the seed makes the spice mace. They both have antibacterial properties. Nutmeg is a warming spice that brings blood from the center of the body to the skin. This action disperses the blood more evenly through the body, reducing overall blood pressure. Myristicin, the active ingredient in the spice, can produce ecstasy-like euphoria, but taking too much can result in nutmeg poisoning. Myristicin inhibits an enzyme in the brain that contributes to Alzheimer's disease and has improved memory in mice in animal studies. Researchers are studying its potential as an antidepressant.

or death

Oregano

Oregano is a powerful antioxidant that reduces inflammation. It contains at least four compounds that soothe coughs and nineteen chemicals with antibacterial action. Oregano is used as a digestive aid.

Parsley

Parsley is a diuretic herb that prevents kidney stones and bladder infections. It increases the production of urine, a property that will support your detox. It contains high levels of chlorophyll that make it effective as a breath freshener. In lab studies, a flavonoid in parsley called apigenin slowed down the growth of prostate cancer cells.

Rosemary

Rosemary improves memory. The ursolic acid in rosemary inhibits the breakdown of a neurotransmitter essential for memory. The herb is rich in antioxidants. Lab studies suggest it may prevent breast cancer and leukemia cells from multiplying. It has been traditionally used to ease asthma and allergy symptoms by reducing the airway constriction induced by histamine.

Saffron

Saffron is the world's most expensive spice. Its brilliant red-orange threads are actually the stigmata from the crocus flower. Saffron contains more than 150 compounds that have antioxidant and antiseptic properties. It has been shown to decrease anxiety and depression. Saffron is believed to promote weight loss by suppressing appetite. In one study, researchers concluded that the antianxiety effect of taking saffron daily may have been what helped overweight women snack about 50 percent less than subjects who took placebos.

Sage

Sage, as its name implies, is a memory enhancer. It protects the brain against processes that lead to Alzheimer's disease. Studies have shown that sage improves mood and increases alertness, calmness, and contentedness. It has anti-inflammatory, antioxidant, and anticancer properties. It may prevent type 2 diabetes and is used to treat diabetes, because it boosts the action of insulin and reduces blood sugar.

Thyme

Thyme has anti-inflammatory properties. By increasing blood flow to the skin, it speeds healing. Thyme is an antispasmodic that eases coughing. The herb is used to treat bronchitis because it relaxes respiratory muscles. The scent of thyme is a mood lifter.

Turmeric

Turmeric gives commercial curry powder its color. It contains the compound curcumin, which has a wide range of benefits. An inflammation fighter, turmeric relieves pain of arthritis and carpal tunnel syndrome. Curcumin is a top anticancer agent. It helps to stop the growth and spread of cancer by reducing the inflammation that contributes to tumor growth. It clears carcinogens away before damage is done to cellular DNA, and can repair damaged DNA. It has been shown to turn off the growth of cancer cells in the colon, pancreas, and skin. Studies have shown that it decreases the formation of amyloid, which is found in deposits in the brains of people with Alzheimer's disease.

Aside from making your food more delicious, your spice rack holds powerful weapons to protect you from harm. Whenever possible, use fresh herbs. Most supermarkets have a great selection. Many detoxers have herb gardens. You can grow herbs in a planter on a deck or terrace, in a small kitchen garden outside, or on your kitchen windowsill, where you can snip off an herb when you need one. Using herbs and spices during your detox will expedite the process of healing.

Fruits

The only fruits you will need on the detox are lemons and limes. You can use slices of these citrus fruits to flavor distilled water. We recommend keeping a pitcher in the refrigerator. You should be drinking at least sixty-four ounces of water a day. Having a pitcher of cool, refreshing flavored water will be appealing. You can also use the fruit slices in iced or hot tea.

Vegetables

When you go to the market to stock up on the vegetables you will be using to make fresh juice, soup, and broth, you should buy about three days' supply of the more delicate leafy greens and plan to use them first. The hardier vegetables—onions, garlic, carrots, sweet potatoes, yams—will retain their nutritional value longer. Greens are an important part of the program, so make sure you have plenty of them. As you are doing your shopping, remember that you are aiming for variety. The list below includes many of the vegetables that are used in our juice and soup recipes.

Garlic
Onions
Leeks
Shallots
Scallions (green onions)
Carrots
Celery
Cucumbers
Fennel
Watercress
Romaine lettuce
Red leaf lettuce
Spinach
Collard greens
Kale
Chard
Dandelion greens
Beet greens
Fresh herbs
White and red cabbage
Brussels sprouts
Asparagus
Green beans
Broccoli
Cauliflower
Beets
Sweet potatoes

Yams
Summer squash
Yellow squash
Zucchini
Acorn squash
Butternut squash

Do your best to buy organic, pesticide-free vegetables for your detox. The purpose of detoxing is to eliminate the toxins that are poisoning you. Eating conventionally grown produce will replace the toxins your body is expelling with new ones. We know that organically raised produce is more expensive, but at least for the month you are devoting to restoring your body, try to be as clean and green as possible. In Chapter 11, Eat Clean, you will find lists of vegetables with low pesticide residue and those with the highest.

You may notice that some of your favorite vegetables are not on the list. Many people are allergic to the nightshade vegetables, specifically eggplant, green, yellow, and red peppers, tomatoes, and white potatoes, without even realizing it. Nightshade vegetables can cause inflammation, a condition you are trying to reduce in your body. A few of the symptoms of a reaction to nightshade vegetables are muscle spasms, pain, and stiffness. During the detox, it is best to stay away from nightshade vegetables. You can introduce them after the detox, but be sensitive to any reactions your body might have.

We are not suggesting that you buy all of the vegetables on this list. Pick and choose according to your taste. Stretch beyond what you usually eat. Flavors will blend in the juice. Be certain that you buy a lot of fresh greens, because they have great healing power and will counter acidity in your body.

When you put your vegetables into the refrigerator, it helps to organize them by color. That way you can be certain you are consuming a rainbow for maximum nutrition. Since you have made shelf space in your cabinets, you can store your supplements within easy reach.

PLANNING YOUR DAY

You want to make doing the detox easy. There are ways to make it work wherever you are. When you are at home, your kitchen is detox central. Your refrigerator is chock-full of fresh vegetables and your vegetable bin is stocked with fresh ginger, cucumbers, and squash. You have your juicer, blender or food processor, and slow cooker lined up on your counter or within easy reach. You have the teakettle ready. You have an adequate supply of distilled water. You are ready to roll.

If you buy individual packets of aloe vera, you might want to keep them on your nightstand or by the bathroom sink to remind you to take that supplement before you go to sleep.

Few of us have the luxury to stay at home during the detox. Many detoxers keep a cooler in their car so that they can make green drinks and fresh juice at home and keep them cold all day. Antioxidant or green drink powders can be mixed in drinking bottles filled with distilled water when you are ready to drink them. In a pinch, you can use a bottle of spring water.

Doing the detox at work might seem like a hassle to you, but if you give it some thought, it is not hard to handle. You can keep the supplements you use during the day in a bowl on your desk or in a drawer. You can store jugs of distilled water under your desk, keeping one in the refrigerator if your office has one.

Juicing at the office may be too much, but there are juice bars everywhere these days. We recommend that you buy freshly squeezed juices, so that you see what goes into them. Many bottled juices are available. Just make certain they are not too sweet, and check the expiration dates. You do not want to drink juice that has been sitting around too long. If finding fresh juice is difficult, you could make your juice before you leave home and bring it in a thermos to keep it cool. A few hours might deplete some nutrients, but

freshly made juice is better than commercially made juices that have a long shelf life. The pasteurized versions of juice you find in the supermarket can be full of preservatives and added sugars. Bottled juices are usually heated at the time of packaging, which kills many of the live raw enzymes. When you buy ready-made juice, study the label. Look for green juice that is sweetened with carrots or beets. Stay away from fruit, including apples. If you cannot find fresh juice and prefer not to bring juice from home, you can substitute your green drink and antioxidant berry drink for your lunchtime juice. Just shake it up in a bottle with eight ounces of distilled water.

It is easy enough to keep a selection of teas at your desk. Most offices have facilities for heating water. If not, you could purchase a small electric kettle or heating coil. You can also bring a thermos of broth to sip from during the workday. If you are working late, soup in a thermos will keep you on your every-two-hour schedule.

> Planning ahead and taking the time to prepare are the keys to a successful detox. I work in an office but do a fair amount of traveling around my city to off-site events and meetings, a light amount of business travel, and have a very busy and active social life. So I am on the go like most Americans. On Sunday of each week, I did the grocery shopping for all of my veggies for my soups and juices. I also scheduled times during the week to prepare my soups. I purchased doubles on the berry drinks and doubles on the green drinks so that I could keep one at home and one at the office. I would make them ahead and put them in a small cooler if I was going to be in the car a lot. I always had a supplement drink before a long meeting, cocktail party, or social outing.
>
> Amy Guerich

SITUATIONAL CHALLENGES

You might find yourself in situations in which you do not have control over what you eat. If you have social engagements, you might not be able to avoid eating at a restaurant or someone else's home. Most chefs today are willing to accommodate you if you call ahead. You can always order simple, steamed vegetables.

If you are invited to a dinner party, you can always tell your host in advance that you are doing a detox and ask if you could bring your own food. Hospitality is about making your guests comfortable. A good host will respect your needs. If you do not want to disrupt your host's plans by bringing your own food or do not want to be conspicuous, eat at home first. At the party, drink a lot of water, take two enzyme pills, eat the vegetables, and move the rest of the food around your plate to make it look as if you have eaten what was served. Close friends and family will already know you are detoxing and will want to support you. Our detoxers tell us that other guests are usually very curious about the program and want to hear all about it.

> The mind is a beautiful thing. Ninety percent of the battle is having the right mind-set. Whether you want your health back or want to lose weight, you have to be committed—so committed that you may have to say no to dinner invites.
>
> I was lucky—friends understood. When a group of us went out to dinner to celebrate a friend's birthday, they were okay with me bringing my juice. I poured it into a glass, ordered a hot tea, brought stevia to sweeten it, and ordered ice water with lots of lemon. Sure, I got a lot of questions, but they saw the transformation, so they were curious.
>
> Kimberly Kirkland Absher

If travel is unavoidable during the month-long detox period, you will have to plan carefully, pack teas and supplements, and look for juice bars and vegetarian or vegan restaurants. Do the best you can. If it is more than a quick trip and you cannot follow the detox as well as you would like, you will slow down your weight loss and diminish the effects of the detox. On your return, you can get with the program and back on track.

*   *   *

The next two chapters cover what foods you are going to eat during your detox. You will learn about juicing and making soups and broths. Both chapters include recipes to help you get the hang of it.

When I had an engagement within the twenty-one days of the detox, I ate before or took my drinks with me, even to a restaurant. While my family ate, I was sticking to my plan. I had the schedule everywhere—in my computers, cell phone, cars, work. I had memorized it in a week, but it's good to have it in sight at all times.

Petrina Devon Young

CHAPTER 6

GET JUICED

Since you are going for high-density nutrition, making your own fresh juice is the perfect delivery system. The more vegetables you eat, the better. Raw vegetables contain important enzymes and micronutrients that heating destroys. If you had to eat all the vegetables you will be juicing on the detox in their whole form, you would face a pile of raw vegetables that almost covers the top of a table and have to do a lot of chewing to put them away. Juicing essentially predigests the vegetables so that your body can absorb the vitamins, minerals, and other nutrients quickly. Fiber is extracted during the juicing process. The presence of fiber in your digestive tract slows down digestion and the absorption of nutrients. When you drink fresh juice, the nutrients in the vegetables are maximally available to the body and quickly flood the bloodstream with their healthy properties, so that healing can take place and more energy is produced for weight loss. Your digestive system also gets a rest.

When you juice, you end up eating a greater variety of vegetables. A square meal usually consists of a protein, a simple carbohydrate, a vegetable, and maybe a salad, which does not bring you close to the number of servings of vegetables you are supposed to be eating in a day. It is so easy to get in a rut and eat the same vegetables and salad every day. When you juice, some vegetables you normally do not eat become more palatable. A glass of freshly made juice can concentrate all the vegetable nutrients recommended for the day or more.

For your convenience, we have created a chart of the vegetables you will be juicing with their vitamin and mineral content as well as their benefits. Use this as a handy reference when you are concocting different combinations for your juices.

VEGETABLE	VITAMIN AND MINERAL CONTENT	BENEFITS
Beets (root and greens)	Vitamin C, iron, calcium, potassium, folate, manganese	Helps to build blood and the immune system. Fights infection. Healing for the liver and gallbladder. Beet juice is a potent juice that should be diluted with cucumber, celery, chard, or another vegetable. Many detoxers use it as a sweetener in their juices.
Broccoli	Vitamins A, C, E, and K; niacin, folate, potassium, calcium, sulfur, indol-3, carbachol, beta-carotene	A powerful antioxidant and energizer, broccoli juice is bitter and should be mixed with sweeter vegetables or lemon juice. Excellent for cleansing; helps fight cancer and cataracts and supports healing.
Cabbage	Vitamin C, beta-carotene, anthocyanins (red cabbage), sulfur	This potent antioxidant fights cancer, heals stomach ulcers, and improves colon conditions.
Carrot	Vitamins A, C, B$_6$; beta-carotene, niacin, folate, pantothenic acid	One of the most powerful antioxidants and detoxifiers. A sweet juice, it can be used to make any combination taste better. Improves eyesight and acne.
Cauliflower	Vitamins A and C, folate, potassium, calcium, magnesium, phosphorus, indol-3	Cauliflower does not yield much juice, but works well in soups. It is a potent cancer-prevention vegetable. Improves digestion and bowel movements, helps build bone, assists blood formation.
Celery	Vitamins A, C, and K; sodium	Celery's high sodium content helps you replenish the sodium you lose while flushing out toxins or sweating.

VEGETABLE	VITAMIN AND MINERAL CONTENT	BENEFITS
Chard	Vitamins A, C, E, and K; potassium, iron, and copper	Prevents digestive tract cancers; has a protective effect on kidneys; helps vision.
Cilantro (Coriander)	Vitamin C, calcium, iron, potassium	Removes heavy metals, like mercury and aluminum, from the body; has antibacterial properties. Tastes great in juice.
Cucumber	Vitamins A, C, and K: manganese, calcium, phosphate, sulfur	Builds blood; aids kidney detox. Very good for eyesight.
Fennel	Vitamins C and E; beta-carotene, iron, manganese, essential fatty acids	Good for digestion; relieves gas.
Garlic	Allicin	Decreases blood pressure and cholesterol; has antibacterial and antimicrobial properties; fights colds and flu; prevents cancer.
Ginger	Vitamin E, selenium, beta-carotene, manganese	Helps relieve nausea; improves metabolism. Ginger has a strong flavor, so watch how much you use; adds great flavor to juice.
Greens (collard, mustard, turnip)	Vitamins A and C; iron calcium, indol-3, potassium, leonine, zeaxanthin	Powerful antioxidants and blood detoxifiers; good for the liver. They help relieve constipation and build blood. They have a strong flavor that many find hard to drink straight. Mix them with carrot, cucumber, or lemon juice.
Kale	Vitamins A, C, and K; folate, potassium	Powerful antioxidant and detoxifier, good for cleansing liver; improves vision.
Onion	Vitamin C, folate, manganese, potassium, phosphate, selenium, allium, allicin, lycopene, anthocyanins	A potent blood purifier. Promotes skin and wound healing.
Parsley	Vitamins A, B_1, B_2, B_3, B_5, K; beta-carotene, calcium, magnesium, phosphorous, iron, potassium, folate, sulfur	Very high in chlorophyll. An antioxidant, it is a blood purifier; aids in detox of the kidney and liver; inhibits tumors, especially in the lung; helps metabolism; contributes to bone health.

VEGETABLE	VITAMIN AND MINERAL CONTENT	BENEFITS
Radish	Folic acid, calcium, potassium	Promotes detoxification and purifies blood.
Spinach	Vitamins A, C, and K; folate, potassium, phosphate, selenium, iron	Spinach is a nutritional powerhouse. A potent antioxidant, it fights inflammation; has cancer-fighting properties, particularly for stomach, prostate, and skin cancers; lowers blood pressure; boosts blood formation and fights anemia; protects eye from cataracts and macular degeneration; boosts immunity; promotes healthy skin; maintains strength and density of bones; fights cardiovascular disease and stroke; promotes healthy nervous system and brain function.
Sweet potato	Vitamins A, C, and B_6; niacin, folate, potassium, phosphate, manganese, selenium, pantothenic acid	Heart-healthy, antioxidant. Helps metabolize carbohydrates; promotes healthy skin and hair.
Turnip	Vitamin C and most B's, calcium, iron, manganese, copper, potassium	Lowers risk of obesity, high blood pressure, diabetes. A powerful antioxidant that detoxifies the liver.

JUICE TIMING

You might be wondering if you could make a pitcher of juice to save time and to avoid cleaning your juicer for a single glass of juice. It is not a good idea. Freshly made juice retains its maximum live nutritional properties for about thirty minutes. After half an hour, the juice begins to oxidize and break down, losing nutrients. Since fresh juice is so perishable, you should try to drink it immediately.

Juice can be stored up to twenty-four hours with moderate nutritional decline if you are careful. Store your juice in a glass jar with an airtight lid. You should fill the jar to the top to reduce the amount of air in the jar. The oxygen in the air will oxidize and deplete your juice of nutrients. Store the jar in the refrigerator immediately.

Dr. Roni's Ten Reasons to Drink Green Juice

There are many reasons green juice improves your health. Green juices restore pH balance, which we will explain in more detail in a later section. To put it simply: toxins, stress, and modern life make your body acidic, and acidity does a lot of damage. It weakens all body systems by producing an internal environment conducive to disease.

Green juices neutralize the acid, bringing your pH balance—the acid-alkaline balance in your interior environment—back to the center, where it is supposed to be. Every time you take a sip of the juice you have made, think of all the good you are doing for your body. Drinking fresh green juice will:

1. Prevent weight gain, diabetes, and obesity. Studies have shown that acidity has considerable influence on weight problems.
2. Prevent corrosion of your arteries, veins, and heart tissue from acidity. When your body is acidic—and most of us are—the acid erodes and eats into cell wall membranes, weakening your heart and circulatory system.
3. Prevent free-radical damage and premature aging. An acidic body accelerates oxidative stress, which destroys cell walls, resulting in wrinkles, age spots, dysfunctional hormonal systems, poor eyesight, and memory loss.
4. Prevent LDL cholesterol plaque from accumulating at an accelerated rate in your blood vessels, clogging up the works.
5. Help to maintain normal blood pressure. When your body is acidic, your arteries can become dilated, making it difficult to control hypertension, arrhythmias, and the advent of heart attacks.
6. Help lipid and fatty acid metabolism. An acidic body disrupts lipid and fatty acid metabolism. Fatty acids are involved in nerve and brain function. When fatty acid metabolism is disturbed, neurological problems may arise, including multiple sclerosis. Hormonal balance is also affected.
7. Help metabolize stored energy reserves. An acidic body interferes with cellular communication, slowing down the processing and absorption of nutrients entering the cells. Green juice returns the body to efficient metabolism.

8. Improve regeneration of cells. For healthy cell proliferation to occur, the body cannot be acidic. Cancerous cells grow well in an acidic environment. When the body is acidic, the possibility of cellular mutations that become cancer accelerates and increases.

9. Get more oxygen to all the cells in the body. An acidic body decreases the amount of oxygen that is delivered to the cells, and this decrease makes normal cells sick.

10. Improve electrolyte function. Electrolytes—potassium, sodium, calcium, and magnesium, for example—are essential for our bodies to function properly. In addition, inhibition of electrolyte activity affects the way we feel and behave, because these minerals give us energy.

JUICE FOR YOUR PALATE

If you are a juicing novice, the taste of primarily green juices could take getting used to. Since you will not be eating processed food or even chewing solid food, the flavors of many raw vegetables might seem very strong to you. Beginners seem to prefer more sweetness in their juices. Using carrots and beets will do the trick. If you are like most detoxers, your palate will change as the benefits kick in. You will become accustomed to the taste of concentrated vegetable flavor. When sweetness is less important, you might flavor your juices with ginger, garlic, parsley, and other herbs. Many people add a teaspoon of fresh lemon juice to their green juice to balance the strong taste of greens.

We have divided our juice recipes into Beginners, Intermediate, and Advanced. The recipes are juices that are served at the Retreat and that we make for ourselves. Many detoxers send us their favorite recipes. We invite you to do the same at our website (www .mvdetoxdiet.com), which links to our Facebook and Twitter pages. Experiment with all sorts of combinations and see what works for you. You do not have to start at the beginners' level. It all depends on what tastes good to you. Remember: the greener your juice, the deeper your detox will be.

What follow are a few of our favorite juices. They are here to give you ideas and to inspire you to come up with new combinations. You will be a juice master sooner than you think.

Before you start, a few reminders on preparing the ingredients:

Scrub all vegetables thoroughly, even those organically grown.

Peel beets, carrots, and garlic, but there is no need to peel ginger or cucumbers.

Trim the stems from green beans and the tough bottoms of asparagus spears and collard greens.

Be sure to include the stems of all leaves and herbs.

BEGINNER JUICES

These recipes are sweet, refreshing, and easy to swallow. Carrots and beets are the natural sweeteners. The green ingredients in these juices are mild. Give them a try.

> During the detox, I would remind myself every day that I was choosing health and not depriving myself of anything. I reminded myself that it was my choice and no one else's. I kept going back to the reason I was doing it. It also helped to remember what Jägermeister tastes like and how I chose to drink that in college. If I could drink that—something that wreaks havoc on the body—I could drink some veggies and treat my body right! I also visualized my body smiling, and oxygen and blood traveling happily through my insides and skin. I think the biggest help was the thought that it was my choice to treat myself like a million dollars as opposed to a five-dollar bill.
>
> Melissa Scarry

CARROT AND GINGER JUICE

6 large carrots
2 cucumbers
1-inch chunk fresh ginger

SWEET SPINACH CARROT JUICE

4 large carrots

2 packed cups spinach

1 small bunch watercress

½-inch slice fresh ginger

1 garlic clove

SWEET IMMUNE JUICE

2 large carrots

1 large beet

1½ cucumbers

GREEN AND ORANGE DELIGHT

5 carrots

1 cup chopped green beans

5 spinach leaves

A TOUCH OF GREEN

5 carrots

4 collard greens

2 parsley sprigs

¼ beet

COOL AND SWEET

1 cucumber

1 beet

3 beet leaves

3 carrots

¼ garlic clove

THE 3 C'S
4 carrots

2 celery stalks

½ head white cabbage

INTERMEDIATE JUICES

At the intermediate level, you will be using fewer sweet ingredients, and will gradually increase the proportion of greens.

POWER PUNCH GREEN JUICE
2 large carrots

1 cucumber

¼ bunch parsley

1 cup chopped green beans

5 Brussels sprouts

CABBAGE, CARROT, AND CAULIFLOWER
½ head red cabbage

3 large carrots

½ cucumber

½ head cauliflower

½ garlic clove

ASPARAGUS DETOX JUICE
1 beet

6 asparagus stalks

1 cucumber

1 garlic clove

HEARTY HEART GREEN JUICE
4 packed cups spinach
1 large bunch watercress
1 carrot
1 cup chopped green beans
½ garlic clove
¼-inch slice fresh ginger

CUCUMBER COLLARD JUICE
1 cucumber
4 collard greens
1 carrot
8 parsley sprigs

GINGER SNAP JUICE
4 broccoli florets
4 spinach leaves
1 carrot
1 cucumber
1-inch piece fresh ginger

SPICY GREEN BEETS JUICE
2 large beets
6 kale leaves
2 celery stalks
10 green beans
¼-inch slice fresh ginger

SQUASH, CELERY, AND CUCUMBER

2 yellow squashes
1 cucumber
1 celery stalk
8 spinach leaves

MAKING THE TRANSITION JUICE

1 cucumber
1 carrot
6 kale leaves
3 collard greens
1 garlic clove

GREEN BEAN JUICE

8 green beans
4 large carrots
4 collard greens
1 garlic clove

STRONG CARROT COMBO

4 carrots
1 celery stalk
6 spinach leaves
6 parsley sprigs
2 garlic cloves

ADVANCED JUICES

When your palate has developed to the advanced level, you will
be juicing a larger proportion of greens and reducing your use of

sweet high-glycemic vegetables. A centrifugal juicer will not get a lot of juice from greens. We use celery and cucumbers to pump up the volume and lemon to balance the strong flavor of greens. Cut the yellow peel and white pith off the lemon and use only the flesh and membranes or just squeeze fresh lemon juice into the juice you have made.

EASY GREEN BEAN JUICE
1 cup chopped green beans
5 spinach leaves
1 cucumber
2 celery stalks
½ lemon

THE GREEN MACHINE
5 spinach leaves
5 kale leaves
5 chard greens
2 celery stalks
1 garlic clove

SUPER 6
6 kale leaves
6 collard greens
6 parsley sprigs
6 broccoli florets
1 celery stalk
½ cucumber

POPEYE SPINACH SPECIAL
12 to 15 spinach leaves
½ cucumber
1 garlic clove

DOWN SOUTH JUICE

1 bunch collard greens
½ cucumber
2 celery stalks
1 garlic clove
1 lemon

MASTER GREEN

5 spinach leaves
5 collard greens
5 watercress sprigs
2 celery stalks
½ lemon
1 garlic clove
¼-inch slice fresh ginger

SUPREME GREEN

1 bunch dandelion greens
5 broccoli florets
2 cucumbers
1 garlic clove
½ lemon

LUCKY 7

7 dandelion greens
7 collard leaves
7 chard leaves
7 spinach leaves
7 kale leaves
1 cucumber
2 celery stalks
1-inch piece fresh ginger

When you drink the juice you have made, you will feel an amazing surge of energy. So many detoxers have told us they are lighter and brighter right away. They experience a vibrancy they thought they had lost forever. That is because their cells are washed in so many vitamins and minerals. Make juicing a part of your life for sustained good health and well-being.

TROUBLESHOOTING CHART

Vegetable juice is good for what ails you. If you have chronic complaints, check out the chart that follows. Common conditions are paired up with the vegetables that will help to correct the problem. Try using vegetables as a remedy to supplement what you are already doing to alleviate whatever is bothering you physically. When you have finished your detox and are on Dr. Roni's Healthy Eating Plan, you will want to refer to this chart to target the effect of the juices you make.

CONDITION	RECOMMENDED VEGETABLE JUICES
Acne	Carrot, cucumber, dandelion greens, endive, fenugreek sprouts, kohlrabi, parsnip, purslane, turnip, turnip greens, wheatgrass
Aging (premature)	Wheatgrass
Anemia	Alfalfa sprouts, asparagus, bean sprouts, beet, beet greens, buckwheat greens, chard, dandelion greens, endive, green beans, kale, kohlrabi, lamb's-quarters, lettuce, parsley, purslane, spinach, turnip, turnip greens, watercress, wheatgrass
Arterial plaque	Buckwheat green
Arthritis	Bean sprouts, bell pepper, carrot, cucumber, fennel, kale, kohlrabi, parsnip, sunflower greens, turnip, turnip greens, wheatgrass
Asthma	Cabbage, cabbage sprouts, carrot, celery, kale, kohlrabi, parsnip, radish, radish sprouts, scallions (green onions), sunflower greens, turnip, turnip greens, wheatgrass
Bladder disorders	Beet, beet greens, cabbage, cabbage sprouts, carrot, dandelion greens, endive, fenugreek sprouts, kohlrabi, parsley, parsnip, purslane, sunflower greens, summer squash, tomato, turnip, turnip greens, watercress, wheatgrass

CONDITION	RECOMMENDED VEGETABLE JUICES
Cough	Scallions (green onions)
Eczema	Cucumber, kohlrabi, radish, radish sprouts
Eye disorders (including cataracts and fatigue)	Alfalfa sprouts, asparagus, beet, beet greens, bell pepper, carrot, dandelion greens, endive, kohlrabi, lamb's-quarters, parsley, parsnip, purslane, sunflower greens, turnip, turnip greens, wheatgrass
Fatigue	Alfalfa sprouts, artichoke, bean sprouts, beet, beet greens, chard, lamb's-quarters, wheatgrass
Female hormone imbalance	Parsley, watercress
Fever	Cucumber
Fluid retention	Bean sprouts, cucumber, fenugreek sprouts
Gout	Asparagus, celery, fennel, tomato
Hair loss	Alfalfa sprouts, bell pepper, cabbage, cabbage sprouts, cucumber, kale, lamb's-quarters, lettuce, watercress, wheatgrass
Hay fever	Carrot, kale, parsnip, wheatgrass
Heart disease	Beet, beet greens, bell pepper, buckwheat greens, dandelion greens, endive, fenugreek sprouts, kohlrabi, parsley, purslane, scallions (green onions), spinach, sunflower greens, turnip, turnip greens
Impotence	Alfalfa sprouts, kale, lamb's-quarters, wheatgrass
Infection	Kohlrabi, scallions (green onions), spinach, turnip, turnip greens, wheatgrass
Insomnia	Celery, lettuce
Intestinal disorders	Alfalfa sprouts, beet, beet greens, carrot, celery, dandelion greens, endive, kale, kohlrabi, lamb's-quarters, lettuce, parsnip, purslane, spinach, sunflower greens, tomato, turnip, turnip greens, watercress, wheatgrass
Jaundice	Beet, beet greens
Kidney disorders	Alfalfa sprouts, asparagus, beet, beet greens, cabbage, cabbage sprouts, celery, cucumber, lamb's-quarters
Liver disorders	Alfalfa sprouts, beet, beet greens, carrot, celery, dandelion greens, endive, kale, kohlrabi, lamb's-quarters, lettuce, parsnip, purslane, spinach, sunflower greens, tomato, turnip, turnip greens, watercress, wheatgrass
Lung disorders	Kohlrabi, sunflower greens, turnip, turnip greens, wheatgrass
Lymph circulation	Beet, beet greens, chard
Malnutrition	Bean sprouts

CONDITION	RECOMMENDED VEGETABLE JUICES
Menopause	Beet, beet greens, chard
Menstrual problems	Beet, beet greens, chard, watercress
Mucus membrane disorders	Beet, beet greens, chard, watercress
Nervous disorders	Asparagus, celery, fennel, lettuce, spinach, wheatgrass
Poor digestion	Spinach
Pregnancy and delivery	Alfalfa sprouts, bean sprouts, beet, beet greens, carrot, chard, kale, lamb's-quarters, parsnip
Prostate disorders	Asparagus, parsley
Psoriasis	Cucumber
Pyorrhea	Cabbage, cabbage sprouts, kale, spinach
Rheumatism	Asparagus
Sinus disorders	Kohlrabi, radish, radish sprouts
Skin disorders	Asparagus, beet, beet greens, bell pepper, carrot, chard, dandelion greens, endive, fenugreek sprouts, green beans, kohlrabi, parsley, parsnip, purslane, radish, radish sprouts, scallions (green onions), spinach, sunflower greens, tomato, turnip, turnip greens, watercress, wheatgrass
Thyroid imbalance	Alfalfa sprouts, cabbage, cabbage sprouts, green beans, kohlrabi, lamb's-quarters, radish, radish sprouts, spinach, watercress
Ulcers	Cabbage, cabbage sprouts, carrot, kale, parsnip, spinach, wheatgrass
Urinary tract infection	Parsley
Weakness (digestive or muscular)	Bean sprouts
Weight (excess)	Alfalfa sprouts, artichoke, bean sprouts, beet, beet greens, buckwheat greens, carrot, celery, cucumber, dandelion greens, endive, fennel, fenugreek sprouts, kale, kohlrabi, lamb's-quarters, lettuce, parsley, parsnip, radish, radish sprouts, scallions (green onions), spinach, sunflower greens, tomato, turnip, turnip greens, watercress, wheatgrass

The other food you will be consuming during your detox is homemade soup. Chapter 7, Clean and Green Soups and Broths, will prepare you to be a soup chef. There is something wonderful about a pot of soup simmering on the stove. It is the ultimate comfort food.

Detox Success Story
IF ANTHONY BOURDAIN HAS BEEN THERE, WE TRY TO GO, TOO

I have done the detox with tremendous results twice. I do, however, fall back into my old ways after. We live in Guam. We are a part of a close expat community. We are very social and are usually at gatherings once to twice a week. I love food and wine, and that is a fun part of our social lives. We also travel quite a bit. We love the cuisine in other cultures. I plan our trips around food adventures. We embrace whatever else may come our way while we travel. If Anthony Bourdain has been there, then we try to go, too.

My life is like so many other women's. I am the mother of two. One of our children has a disability, which requires extra therapy every week on top of the sports and academic activities that keep me on the go. All this starts to run me down. I feel sluggish, things become ill fitting, and I begin to feel the need to give myself a "gift" and do another full detox.

It's hard! I won't lie. It requires planning—I live in Guam, where nothing is available. I actually keep all the stuff on hand in my cabinet for when I feel I need a day or two to just clean things up a bit. I stock up whenever I visit back in the States. My biggest struggle is the social activities. I limit them while I detox, because the wine is such a temptation. However, it is all worth it.

My body looks amazing, feels amazing, and quite frankly, my husband loves that I become even more attentive to him because I feel so good. He has done the detox with me, which makes it even easier, and he has loved the results, too. He is at Oktoberfest with friends right now and has already e-mailed home to say that he wants to get back on the wagon when he gets back. So there you have it. I'm just a normal person who goes on and off the diet every six months to a year.

Kim Eby Bruch

CHAPTER 7

CLEAN AND GREEN SOUPS AND BROTHS

Your dinner on the detox will be a rich and delicious vegetable soup, although you will not be eating the vegetables whole. You will remove the vegetables from the soup and puree them in a blender or food processor. The master soup recipe does not take major kitchen skills. Even if you are not much of a cook, making these soups is a breeze. Pretend you are on a cook-off on the Food Network as you create your soup. This is all it takes.

You can use any combination of vegetables you would like from the list starting on page 109. Some vegetables on the list do better in soup than in juice: cauliflower, sweet potatoes, and yams add body. Carrots, squash, sweet potatoes, yams, and beets add sweetness. Make the broth flavorful by adding garlic, onions, dill, parsley, bay leaf, or no-salt vegetable seasoning. Broth will keep up to three days if refrigerated. You can make a large quantity and freeze it in individual portions. Any of the soups you make will be more flavorful if you use vegetable broth instead of water. Make a big pot of broth so that you can use it for making soup.

James's rule of thumb is that a gallon plastic bag filled with vegetables with a gallon of distilled water makes two portions of soup and extra broth. The idea, just as with your juicing, is to increase the quantity of greens you eat. Just eyeball the proportion of vegetables that looks right to you as you toss them into a pot of distilled water. You cannot really make a mistake. The vegetables are going to be pureed in the end. Make sure the water is a few inches above the vegetables. Bring the water to a boil and cook for 15 to 30 minutes, depending on how hard the vegetables are. If you can pierce them with a fork, they are ready.

MASTER SOUP

About 2 cups soup and 1½ quarts broth

1. In a large pot, combine 2 quarts distilled water and 2 cups trimmed, cut-up vegetables. Add your favorite herbs and spices.

2. Bring to a boil over high heat. Lower the heat and simmer for 10 to 20 minutes, until all the vegetables are soft. When you can stick a fork in the vegetables, they are ready.

3. Place a large fine-mesh strainer over a large clean storage container. Carefully pour in the soup, collecting the vegetables in the strainer and the broth in the storage container.

4. Transfer the vegetables to a blender or food processor. Add ¼ to ½ cup of the broth, cover, and puree until smooth. Be careful, as the soup will be hot. Add more broth if you like the soup thinner.

5. Eat the soup right away, or transfer it to a separate container, let it cool to room temperature, cover, and refrigerate. Reheat over low heat when needed. Let the remaining broth cool, cover, and refrigerate until needed.

Keep the broth to drink during the day. A cup of broth equals a cup of water. It counts toward your water intake, but it is much tastier.

Save the scraps left over from cutting up the vegetables for your juice and soup. You can throw them along with other vegetables and seasonings into a slow cooker filled with distilled water to make a broth you can drink all day. Drinking broth can take the edge off hunger. At the Martha's Vineyard Holistic Retreat, we call this Free Soup. The calories in the broth are offset by the number of calories your body uses to digest the broth.

FREE SOUP

4 to 5 cups

1. In a medium pot or small slow cooker, combine 1 quart distilled water and 2 cups trimmed, cut-up vegetables of your choice. Onions, carrots, and celery make a good base. Do not forget the greens. Add your favorite herbs and spices.

2. If using the stove, bring to a boil over high heat. Lower the heat and simmer for 30 to 60 minutes. If using a slow cooker, cover and cook on low all day.

3. Remove the vegetables with a slotted spoon.

4. If you really want to indulge and add more body to the broth, puree 1 cup of the vegetables in a blender or food processor. Add a little of the broth, if necessary. Stir back into the pot of broth. Discard any remaining vegetables.

5. Cover the pot or slow cooker and keep the broth warm on the lowest possible heat. Be sure to stir it before ladling out a portion.

You can season the soup to taste. If you are not used to using herbs and spices, be conservative. You can always add more. If you are heavy-handed, just add more water to dilute the flavor.

We thought it might be helpful to give you some ideas about combining herbs and spices. Herbs are green leaves and spices are seeds, roots, bark, and berries. The stronger the taste of the seasoning you are using, the less you should use. Rule of thumb: add herbs and spices the last fifteen to twenty minutes of cooking.

The ethnic combinations that follow are classics. Experiment and create your own favorites.

> **Protein Boost**
>
> Bragg Liquid Aminos is a liquid protein made from non–genetically modified soybeans and purified water. It contains sixteen essential and nonessential amino acids, the building blocks of protein. Feel free to add a tablespoon or so to your soups and broths. On Dr. Roni's Healthy Eating Plan maintenance, you might want to use it like soy sauce on salads and vegetables.

Southern: Cayenne, garlic, coriander, cumin, bay leaves, cilantro

Mediterranean: basil, bay leaves, oregano, thyme or rosemary, garlic

Herbes de Provence: basil, chervil, fennel, lavender, marjoram, rosemary, savory, tarragon, thyme

Mexican: Chili powder, cumin, oregano, cayenne

Indian #1: cumin, coriander, cilantro, garlic, ginger, cayenne

Indian #2: curry or garam masala, turmeric, garlic, ginger, cayenne

Middle Eastern #1: cumin, coriander, chili

Middle Eastern #2: cumin, coriander, ginger

Middle Eastern #3: cinnamon, coriander, ginger

For those of you who would rather follow a recipe than go freestyle, we have provided some exceptional soup recipes you are sure to enjoy. When you sit down to have your soup, you can drink some hot broth from the pot or a cup of hot tea after you eat. You can make a big pot of soup and freeze individual portions.

If a vegetable is not listed as "peeled," there is no need to peel it.

Onions, garlic, beets, carrots, turnips, and winter squashes should always be peeled. Just be sure to scrub or rinse other vegetables well.

Dried Herb to Fresh Herb Conversion

If you are using dried herbs, you need to use less than fresh herbs. Generally speaking, this is the formula:

1 teaspoon of dry herbs = 1 tablespoon of fresh herbs

Try to use fresh herbs whenever you can.

GROUP SOUP

6 servings

2 quarts distilled water
4 carrots, peeled and chopped
2 turnips, peeled and chopped
2 zucchini, chopped
2 leeks (roots and any bruised dark-green leaves removed), chopped and thoroughly rinsed to remove all grit
1 onion, peeled and chopped
2 celery stalks, chopped
1 medium head white cabbage, quartered, cored, and chopped
4 bay leaves
1 whole head garlic, separated into cloves and peeled
20 parsley sprigs
¼ cup no-salt vegetable seasoning
1 teaspoon cayenne pepper (if you like it spicier, add more to taste)

1. Combine all the ingredients in a large pot and bring to a boil over high heat. Reduce the heat to medium, cover, and simmer for about 30 minutes, stirring from time to time, until all the vegetables are tender.

2. Place a large fine-mesh strainer over a large clean container. Carefully pour in the soup, collecting the vegetables in the strainer and the broth in the container. Remove and discard the bay leaves.

3. Working in batches if necessary, transfer the vegetables to a blender or food processor. Add ¼ to ½ cup of the broth and puree until smooth. Be careful, as the soup will be hot. Do not overfill the food processor or blender. Add more broth if you like the soup thinner.

4. Set aside one-sixth of the soup for your dinner portion. Refrigerate or freeze the remaining soup for later use.

5. Divide the remaining broth among storage containers. Let the broth cool to room temperature. Cover and refrigerate or freeze for later use.

RED SOUP

4 servings

2 quarts distilled water
½ cup chopped peeled beets
½ cup chopped peeled carrots
¼ cup fresh sage leaves
3 cups chopped red cabbage

1. Combine the water, beets, carrots, and sage in a large pot. Bring to a boil over high heat. Cook for about 15 minutes, until the beets and carrots are barely tender.

2. Add the cabbage and cook for another 10 minutes, until all the vegetables are soft.

3. Remove the vegetables with a slotted spoon. Transfer the vegetables to a blender or food processor. Add ¼ to ½ cup of

the broth and puree until smooth. Be careful, as the soup will be hot. Do not overfill the food processor or blender. Add more broth if you like the soup thinner.

4. Set aside one-quarter of the soup for your dinner portion. Refrigerate or freeze the remaining soup for later use.

5. Divide the remaining broth among storage containers. Let the broth cool to room temperature. Cover and refrigerate or freeze for later use.

A VARIATION ON RED CABBAGE SOUP

6 servings

1 gallon unsalted vegetable broth or distilled water
2 heads red cabbage, quartered, cored, and chopped
1 large Vidalia onion, peeled and chopped
1 cup chopped celery
1 large sweet potato, chopped
½ bunch parsley
3 tablespoons fresh thyme leaves or 1 tablespoon dried
1 tablespoon fresh marjoram leaves or 1 teaspoon dried
1 teaspoon cayenne pepper, or more to taste

1. Combine all the ingredients in a large pot and bring to a boil over high heat. Reduce the heat to medium, cover, and simmer for 15 to 20 minutes, until the vegetables are very soft.

2. Place a large fine-mesh strainer over a large clean container. Carefully pour in the soup, collecting the vegetables in the strainer and the broth in the container.

3. Working in batches if necessary, transfer the vegetables to a blender or food processor. Add ¼ to ½ cup of the broth and puree until smooth. Be careful, as the soup will be hot. Do not

overfill the food processor or blender. Add more broth if you like the soup thinner.

4. Set aside one-sixth of the soup for your dinner portion. Refrigerate or freeze the remaining soup for later use, if you like.

5. Divide the remaining broth among storage containers. Let the broth cool to room temperature. Cover and refrigerate or freeze for later use.

GREEN LEEK SOUP

This soup is very spicy, and good to replace minerals after sweating.

4 servings

1 quart distilled water
2 onions, peeled and chopped
3 carrots, peeled and chopped
6 celery stalks, chopped
1 leek (with dark-green leaves removed), chopped and
    thoroughly rinsed to remove all grit
1 cup chopped fresh spinach
½ head white cabbage, cored and chopped
¼ cup Bragg Liquid Aminos
Leaves from 2 thyme sprigs
Leaves from 1 sage sprig, chopped
Leaves from 2 basil sprigs, chopped
2 teaspoons cayenne pepper

1. Combine the water, onions, carrots, celery, leek, spinach, and cabbage in a large pot and bring to a boil over high heat. Reduce the heat to medium and simmer for 15 to 20 minutes, until the vegetables are tender.

2. Place a large fine-mesh strainer over a large clean container. Carefully pour in the soup, collecting the vegetables in the strainer and the broth in the container.

3. Working in batches if necessary, transfer the vegetables to a blender or food processor. Add the liquid aminos, thyme, sage, basil, and cayenne. Add ¼ to ½ cup of the broth and puree until smooth. Be careful, as the soup will be hot. Do not overfill the food processor or blender. Add more broth if you like the soup thinner.

4. Set aside one-quarter of the soup for your dinner portion. Refrigerate or freeze the remaining soup for later use.

5. Divide the remaining broth among storage containers. Let the broth cool to room temperature. Cover and refrigerate or freeze for later use.

SWEET PARSNIP SOUP

4 servings

6 cups unsalted vegetable broth or distilled water
6 parsnips, peeled and chopped
2 sweet potatoes, chopped
1 large onion, peeled and chopped
2 leeks (roots and any bruised dark-green leaves removed),
    chopped and thoroughly rinsed to remove all grit
3 tablespoons fresh lemon juice
⅛ teaspoon cayenne pepper

1. Combine all the ingredients in a large pot and bring to a boil over high heat. Reduce the heat to medium, cover, and simmer for 15 to 20 minutes, until all the vegetables are tender.

2. Place a large fine-mesh strainer over a large clean container. Carefully pour in the soup, collecting the vegetables in the strainer and the broth in the container.

3. Working in batches if necessary, transfer the vegetables to a blender or food processor. Add ¼ to ½ cup of the broth and puree until smooth. Be careful, as the soup will be hot. Do not overfill the food processor or blender. Add more broth if you like the soup thinner.

4. Set aside one-quarter of the soup for your dinner portion. Refrigerate or freeze the remaining soup for later use.

5. Divide the remaining broth among storage containers. Let the broth cool to room temperature. Cover and refrigerate or freeze for later use.

FAMILY GARDEN SOUP

8 servings

2 quarts unsalted vegetable broth or distilled water
¾ cup chopped onion
2 garlic cloves, chopped
3 sweet potatoes, peeled and chopped
4 celery stalks, sliced
1 carrot, peeled and chopped
2 cups chopped white cabbage
2 acorn squashes or 1 medium butternut squash, peeled, seeded, and chopped
2 medium zucchini, chopped
2 bay leaves
1 tablespoon chili powder
½ teaspoon cayenne pepper

¼ teaspoon ground allspice
¼ teaspoon ground cloves

1. Combine all the ingredients in a large pot and bring to a boil over high heat. Reduce the heat to medium, cover, and simmer for 20 to 30 minutes, until all the vegetables are tender.

2. Place a large fine-mesh strainer over a large clean container. Carefully pour in the soup, collecting the vegetables in the strainer and the broth in the container. Remove and discard the bay leaves.

3. Working in batches if necessary, transfer the vegetables to a blender or food processor. Add ¼ to ½ cup of the broth and puree until smooth. Be careful, as the soup will be hot. Do not overfill the food processor or blender. Add more broth if you like the soup thinner.

4. Set aside one-eighth of the soup for your dinner portion. Refrigerate or freeze the remaining soup for later use.

5. Divide the remaining broth among storage containers. Let the broth cool to room temperature. Cover and refrigerate or freeze for later use.

CREAMY CAULIFLOWER BROCCOLI SOUP

2 servings

6 cups unsalted vegetable broth or distilled water
1 cup cauliflower florets
1 teaspoon chopped fresh oregano
2 garlic cloves, peeled and chopped
A few parsley sprigs, chopped

2 cups broccoli florets
1 cup chopped green beans
1 cup chopped peeled carrots
No-salt vegetable seasoning (optional)

1. Combine 2 cups of the broth or water, the cauliflower, oregano, garlic, and parsley in a small pot. Bring to a boil over high heat. Reduce the heat to medium and simmer until the cauliflower is very soft, about 20 minutes.

2. Place a medium fine-mesh strainer over a clean container. Carefully pour in the cauliflower, collecting the solids in the strainer and the broth in the container. Transfer the cauliflower to a blender or food processor. Add just enough of its broth to be able to puree it, and puree until smooth. Set the cauliflower cream aside, keeping it warm. Rinse out the blender.

3. Combine the remaining cauliflower broth and vegetable broth, the broccoli, green beans, and carrots in a medium pot. Bring to a boil over high heat. Reduce the heat to medium and simmer until the vegetables are tender, 15 to 20 minutes.

4. Remove the vegetables with a slotted spoon and transfer to the blender. Add about 2 tablespoons of the broth and puree until smooth and thick. Season to taste with the vegetable seasoning, if desired.

5. Divide the soup between two serving bowls. Top with the cauliflower cream and serve immediately.

6. Divide the remaining broth among storage containers. Let the broth cool to room temperature. Cover and refrigerate or freeze for later use.

HOLIDAY FEAST SOUP

4 servings

1 quart unsalted vegetable broth or distilled water
2 leeks (roots and any bruised dark-green leaves removed),
   chopped and thoroughly rinsed to remove all grit, or
   2 onions, peeled and chopped
5 medium carrots, peeled and chopped
1 large turnip, peeled and chopped
2 sweet potatoes, chopped
½ medium head white cabbage, cored and chopped
1 teaspoon no-salt vegetable seasoning
Fennel leaves, for garnish

1. Combine the broth or water, leeks, carrots, turnip, sweet potatoes, cabbage, and vegetable seasoning in a large pot. Bring to a boil over high heat. Turn off the heat, cover, and let rest for 15 to 20 minutes.

2. Bring back to a boil. Reduce the heat to low, cover, and simmer for 15 minutes, stirring from time to time, until all the vegetables are soft.

3. Place a large fine-mesh strainer over a large clean container. Carefully pour in the soup, collecting the vegetables in the strainer and the broth in the container.

4. Working in batches if necessary, transfer the vegetables to a blender or food processor. Add ¼ to ½ cup of the broth and puree until creamy and smooth. Be careful, as the soup will be hot. Do not overfill the food processor or blender. Add more broth if you like the soup thinner.

5. Set aside one-quarter of the soup for your dinner portion. Refrigerate or freeze the remaining soup for later use.

6. Divide the remaining broth among storage containers. Let the broth cool to room temperature. Cover and refrigerate or freeze for later use.

7. Gently reheat the soup over low heat and serve hot, garnished with fennel leaves.

GINGER CARROT SOUP

2 servings

1 quart unsalted vegetable broth or distilled water
1 cup chopped peeled carrots
1 cup chopped celery
½ cup chopped sweet potatoes
½-inch slice peeled fresh ginger, finely chopped
1 teaspoon ground cinnamon
1 teaspoon ground cloves
1 teaspoon ground nutmeg
1 teaspoon organic vanilla extract
1 teaspoon stevia

1. Combine the broth or water, carrots, celery, sweet potatoes, ginger, cinnamon, cloves, and nutmeg in a medium pot. Bring to a boil over high heat. Reduce the heat to medium and simmer until the vegetables are tender, 15 to 20 minutes.

2. Remove the vegetables with a slotted spoon and transfer to a blender or food processor. Add ¼ cup of the broth and puree until smooth. Add the vanilla and stevia and blend briefly to combine.

3. Set aside one-half of the soup for your dinner portion. Refrigerate or freeze the remaining soup for later use.

4. Divide the remaining broth among storage containers. Let the broth cool to room temperature. Cover and refrigerate or freeze for later use.

SPICED CARROT-GREEN SOUP

4 servings

4 quarts unsalted vegetable broth
1 quart distilled water
18 carrots, peeled and chopped
2 packed cups spinach
1½ heads romaine lettuce, chopped
2 large sweet potatoes, chopped
2 teaspoons chopped peeled fresh ginger
1 teaspoon ground cinnamon
1 teaspoon ground cloves
1 teaspoon ground nutmeg
1 teaspoon stevia
2 teaspoons organic vanilla extract

1. Combine the broth, water, carrots, spinach, lettuce, sweet potatoes, ginger, cinnamon, cloves, nutmeg, and stevia in a large pot and bring to a boil over high heat. Reduce the heat to medium and simmer for 20 to 30 minutes, until the vegetables are tender.

2. Place a large fine-mesh strainer over a large clean container. Carefully pour in the soup, collecting the vegetables in the strainer and the broth in the container.

3. Working in batches if necessary, transfer the vegetables to a blender or food processor. Add the vanilla. Add ¼ to ½ cup of the broth and puree until smooth. Be careful, as the soup will be hot. Do not overfill the food processor or blender. Add more broth if you like the soup thinner.

4. Set aside one-quarter of the soup for your dinner portion. Refrigerate or freeze the remaining soup for later use.

5. Divide the remaining broth among storage containers. Let the broth cool to room temperature. Cover and refrigerate or freeze for later use.

"STIR-FRY" BROCCOLI SOUP

4 servings

2 quarts distilled water
1 cup chopped peeled carrots
2 cups broccoli florets, chopped
2 cups chopped green beans
1 extra-large Vidalia onion, peeled and chopped
1 head red leaf lettuce
1 tablespoon chopped peeled garlic
1 teaspoon no-salt vegetable seasoning
1 teaspoon stevia

1. Combine all the ingredients in a large pot and bring to a boil over high heat. Reduce the heat to medium, cover, and simmer for 15 to 20 minutes, until the vegetables are tender.

2. Place a large fine-mesh strainer over a large clean container. Carefully pour in the soup, collecting the vegetables in the strainer and the broth in the container.

3. Working in batches if necessary, transfer the vegetables to a blender or food processor. Add ¼ to ½ cup of the broth and puree until smooth. Be careful, as the soup will be hot. Do not overfill the food processor or blender. Add more broth if you like the soup thinner. Set aside one-quarter of the soup for your dinner portion. Refrigerate or freeze the remaining soup for later use.

4. Divide the remaining broth among storage containers. Let the broth cool to room temperature. Cover and refrigerate or freeze for later use.

PUMPKIN SOUP

4 servings

6 cups unsalted vegetable broth or distilled water
5 cups chopped peeled pumpkin or winter squash
2 sweet potatoes, chopped
2 carrots, peeled and chopped
2 garlic cloves, peeled and chopped
½ cup chopped parsley
2 tablespoons organic vanilla extract
1 teaspoon ground nutmeg
1 teaspoon ground cinnamon
1 teaspoon ground cloves
1 teaspoon ground ginger
¼ teaspoon stevia

1. Combine the broth or water, pumpkin, sweet potatoes, carrots, and garlic in a large pot and bring to a boil over high heat. Reduce the heat to medium, cover, and simmer for 20 to 30 minutes, until all the vegetables are tender.

2. Place a large fine-mesh strainer over a large clean container. Carefully pour in the soup, collecting the vegetables in the strainer and the broth in the container.

3. Working in batches if necessary, transfer the vegetables to a blender or food processor. Add the parsley, vanilla, nutmeg, cinnamon, cloves, ginger, and stevia. Add ¼ to ½ cup of the broth and puree until smooth. Be careful, as the soup will be hot. Do not overfill the food processor or blender. Add more broth if you like the soup thinner.

4. Set aside one-quarter of the soup for your dinner portion. Refrigerate or freeze the remaining soup for later use.

5. Divide the remaining broth among five storage containers. Let the broth cool to room temperature. Cover and refrigerate or freeze for later use.

ASIAN SPINACH SOUP

4 servings

1 quart distilled water or unsalted vegetable broth
3 packed cups spinach
1 cup chopped chard
½ cup green beans, cut in half
1 teaspoon Asian chili sauce
2 garlic cloves, peeled
1 tablespoon Bragg Liquid Aminos
½-inch piece fresh ginger

1. Combine all the ingredients in a large pot and bring to a boil over high heat. Reduce the heat to medium, cover, and simmer for 15 to 20 minutes, until the vegetables are tender.

2. Place a large fine-mesh strainer over a large clean container. Carefully pour in the soup, collecting the vegetables in the strainer and the broth in the container.

3. Working in batches if necessary, transfer the vegetables to a blender or food processor. Add ¼ to ½ cup of the broth and puree until smooth. Be careful, as the soup will be hot. Do not overfill the food processor or blender. Add more broth if you like the soup thinner.

4. Set aside one-quarter of the soup for your dinner portion. Refrigerate or freeze the remaining soup for later use.

5. Divide the remaining broth among five storage containers. Let the broth cool to room temperature. Cover and refrigerate or freeze for later use.

MUSTARD AND COLLARD GREENS SOUP

4 servings

3 quarts unsalted vegetable broth
1 bunch mustard greens, chopped (about 2 cups)
1 bunch collard greens, chopped (about 2 cups)
1 large onion, peeled and chopped
4 large carrots, peeled and chopped
2 tablespoons Bragg Liquid Aminos
2 teaspoons chopped peeled fresh ginger

1. Combine all the ingredients in a large pot and bring to a boil over high heat. Reduce the heat to medium; cover; and simmer for 20 to 30 minutes, until the vegetables are tender.

2. Place a large fine-mesh strainer over a large clean container. Carefully pour in the soup, collecting the vegetables in the strainer and the broth in the container.

3. Working in batches if necessary, transfer the vegetables to a blender or food processor. Add ¼ to ½ cup of the broth and puree until smooth. Be careful, as the soup will be hot. Do not overfill the food processor or blender. Add more broth if you like the soup thinner.

4. Set aside one-quarter of the soup for your dinner portion. Refrigerate or freeze the remaining soup for later use.

5. Divide the remaining broth among storage containers. Let the broth cool to room temperature. Cover and refrigerate or freeze for later use.

SWEET CABBAGE SOUP

4 servings

3 quarts unsalted vegetable broth or distilled water
½ head white cabbage, cored and chopped
2 onions, peeled and chopped
2 celery stalks, chopped
2 sweet potatoes, chopped
2 garlic cloves, peeled and chopped
1 bay leaf
½ teaspoon dried basil
½ teaspoon dried thyme

1. Combine the broth or water, cabbage, onions, celery, sweet potatoes, garlic, and bay leaf in a large pot and bring to a boil over high heat. Reduce the heat to medium, cover, and simmer for 15 to 20 minutes, until the vegetables are tender.

2. Add the basil and thyme and simmer for 5 minutes more.

3. Place a large fine-mesh strainer over a large clean container. Carefully pour in the soup, collecting the vegetables in the strainer and the broth in the container. Remove the bay leaf.

4. Working in batches if necessary, transfer the vegetables to a blender or food processor. Add ¼ to ½ cup of the broth and puree until smooth. Be careful, as the soup will be hot. Do not overfill the food processor or blender. Add more broth if you like the soup thinner.

5. Set aside one-quarter of the soup for your dinner portion. Refrigerate or freeze the remaining soup for later use.

6. Divide the remaining broth among storage containers. Let the broth cool to room temperature. Cover and refrigerate or freeze for later use.

CURRIED VEGETABLE SOUP

4 servings

1 quart distilled water or unsalted vegetable broth
1 cup chopped peeled carrots
1 cup chopped collard greens
1 cup chopped yellow squash
1 cup chopped green beans
1 scallion (green onion), trimmed and chopped
4 garlic cloves, peeled
1 teaspoon curry powder
1 teaspoon ground turmeric
1 teaspoon ground cinnamon
1 teaspoon ground nutmeg
1 teaspoon ground ginger
1 teaspoon cayenne pepper

1. Combine all the ingredients in a large pot and bring to a boil over high heat. Reduce the heat to medium; cover; and simmer for 20 to 30 minutes, until the vegetables are tender.

2. Taste the broth. If you find it too spicy, add more water.

3. Place a large fine-mesh strainer over a large clean container. Carefully pour in the soup, collecting the vegetables in the strainer and the broth in the container.

4. Working in batches if necessary, transfer the vegetables to a blender or food processor. Add ¼ to ½ cup of the broth and puree until smooth. Be careful, as the soup will be hot. Do not

overfill the food processor or blender. Add more broth if you like the soup thinner.

5. Set aside one-quarter of the soup for your dinner portion. Refrigerate or freeze the remaining soup for later use.

6. Divide the remaining broth among storage containers. Let the broth cool to room temperature. Cover and refrigerate or freeze for later use.

*   *   *

Don't these soups sound delicious? With no sugar, salt, or other synthetic additives, the soups will give you a new appreciation of subtle, natural flavor. You can prepare them for the shift in your eating habits after the detox. The smell of homemade soup is so wonderful that your family and friends will be curious about what is cooking on the back burner or in the slow cooker. When they see how you change day by day during your detox month, they might be inspired to follow in your footsteps.

Many detoxers incorporate broths and soups into their everyday eating after completing the program to keep their vegetable intake high. Why just drink water when you can bathe your cells with the vitamins and minerals from the broth you make?

Now you have your marching orders. You know what you have to do to lose 1 pound a day and get rid of those toxins that are weighing you down in every respect. The following chapter will describe a number of things you can do to deepen your detox and make it go more smoothly. We will begin by explaining the "healing crisis" that many detoxers experience between days three and seven as toxins begin to be released.

Detox Success Story
WHAT ARE YOU DOING TO LOOK THIS WAY?

I have known James Hester for more than fifteen years. We worked together back in the day. Those times were crazy, stressful, and very toxic.

I remember the day James called me as if it were yesterday. He told me about his life-changing detox in Martha's Vineyard with Dr. Roni DeLuz. I hadn't spoken with James in about a year, but I could tell by his voice that he had experienced something very special and really transforming. I remember him saying, "Jackie, you need to do this detox! I know you have been going through some stressful times and are feeling very broken right now. Listen to me, doing this detox will change you. Not only in a physical way, but also mentally and spiritually!"

Even though I could tell James was a different person, happier, lighter, and full of energy, I just wasn't quite ready to take the plunge and go down the path of being healthy. I think I was scared. I had been unhealthy for so many years, it was the way my body was used to being and feeling. I had become accustomed to being unhealthy.

From time to time James would call to check in and see how I was doing. With every phone call, he asked, "Jackie, have you read the book? You should do the detox."

Every time I would say, "Yes, I know." Once the called ended, I could not take the first step.

This went on for about a year and a half. My health was worsening. My life consisted of insomnia, high blood pressure, hot flashes, night sweats, and anxiety. I was addicted to Ambien to get a decent night's sleep, taking blood pressure and antianxiety pills, and trying conventional and nonconventional methods for my perimenopause. Just like clockwork, James called to ask me if I could come up to the Vineyard to help him do some administrative work and organize his office for him.

Secretly, while James was on the phone, I kept thinking, "Hope he will ask me if I want to do the detox with him when I am up in the Vineyard." I knew my life could not continue at this pace. I felt sluggish, tired, and not like my old self—the happy-go-lucky person I knew I really was. And I weighed the most I ever weighed in my life—a whopping 150 pounds. I normally weigh 123 to 130.

My prayers were answered! James asked me if I wanted to do the detox with him. Before he could even finish asking, a big YES came out of my mouth. I knew then and there that something special was going to begin to transform my life forever! And it did.

I embarked on my first detox in May 2009. I lost only sixteen pounds, owing to hormonal issues, but that was not my main reason for doing the detox. When I completed the detox, I no longer needed Ambien to get a good night's rest; my hot flashes had disappeared, and waking up in the middle of the night drenched in sweat was a thing of the past. My blood pressure was normal. Most important, I no longer needed my antianxiety medication.

When I came back from the Vineyard, my friends almost didn't recognize me. Not only had I changed physically, but my energy was lighter, my skin was glowing, my hair was shiny, and I just couldn't stop smiling. Even strangers picked up on this new and wonderful energy I was exuding. When I went to the doctor to get my annual exam, she couldn't believe how wonderful I looked and how all my test results had changed for the better.

Since I did want to lose more weight, I did a seven-day detox and lost a pound a day. I have made the detox program a part of my life. I am proud to say that I lead a healthy lifestyle. A few things changed in my diet that I didn't expect. For one thing, I was a steak girl—had to have steak at least three or four times a week. With no conscious effort on my part, my body took over and didn't crave steak or red meat anymore. I used to gag on many vegetables and stayed away from them. Those are now my favorite vegetables, and I just can't get enough of them.

I met up with an old girlfriend. We hadn't seen each other in twenty years. When my girlfriend saw me, she said, "Wow! Jacqueline, you look great and haven't changed! What are you doing to look this way?" With much love and pride, I told her my detox story. She is getting ready to start her first detox.

Words cannot begin to express how James and Dr. Roni changed my life—and in many ways, saved it.

Jacqueline Malloy

CHAPTER 8

CRANK UP YOUR HEALING

If you follow the plan described in the previous chapters, you will lose weight and lower your body burden, but you can go a step further if you choose. At the Martha's Vineyard Holistic Retreat, we support the program with therapeutic detoxifying body treatments. In this chapter, we will describe a number of techniques you can do at home that will help your body power through the toxic elimination process and lift the level of your healing. Our techniques include mild exercise, skin brushing for lymphatic drainage, detoxifying baths, and even an at-home body wrap if you can stand the mess. We will also suggest some treatments that require professional help.

1 Pound a Day will live up to its promise even if you do not do anything you find in this chapter and simply follow the eating plan. But while you are focused on detoxing, doesn't it make sense to give your body all the help it can get? By doing a few simple things, you can boost the effectiveness of the detox. At the end of the chapter, we will do some troubleshooting and give you some tips for speeding up your weight loss if it slows down.

As we have mentioned earlier, many detoxers experience what we refer to as a healing crisis, the physical reaction that takes place when your cells expel toxins into the bloodstream and organs more quickly than the body releases them. Headaches are among the most common symptom. Not everyone has a healing crisis. Fifty percent of detoxers experience one at the retreat, mostly because they have chronic illnesses. Though you might skip the healing crisis completely, we did want to warn you that you might feel less than great shortly after starting. If you do have a healing crisis, look on the bright side: consider it a sign that your body has begun to release toxins. This chapter will give you ways to speed your recovery.

THE HEALING CRISIS

Do not be surprised if you feel off between days three and seven of the detox. Your cells are dumping toxic residues into your bloodstream and organs more quickly than your body can eliminate them. That can make you feel unwell. Your body is changing over from acidic food, toxins, preservatives, chemicals, and excess salt and sugar to green drinks, antioxidants, and enzyme-rich, healthy foods. This is a big change. While your body is reacting to the flood of toxins being released, it is adjusting to receiving such healthy, dense nutrients. Some—but not all—detoxers have a healing crisis before the building and restoration begins. We like to call it a healing opportunity.

The sudden release of so many toxins can have physical, emotional, and spiritual effects. The intensity and duration of your crisis depend on how toxic you are and how quickly your body is unloading. Many detoxers feel as if they have a mild flu. You may experience headaches, chills, nausea, fatigue, body aches, constipation, diarrhea, vomiting, cold sores, runny nose, acne, rashes, and ear problems. You might feel worse than when you

> I do believe my body was going through a healing crisis over the past couple days as I just feel bad . . . My stomach was rumbling a lot yesterday, so maybe that is where the work was happening. Anyway, today I feel great! I feel a sense of peace and calm. No stomach rumbling, no hungriness, no cravings.
>
> Tiffany Rogers

started the detox. This will pass in a day or two. Detoxers who have a chronic illness sometimes take up to a week to work through the healing crisis. Remember: the healing crisis is a sign that something good is happening. You will soon be over the hump.

Your cells resist change. As you remember from the discussion of obesogens, your body wants to hold on to the toxins that are stored in your fat cells. Those toxins are stored to protect you, to keep them from damaging your organs and other tissues. When your body releases those toxins, you can feel it. At the same time, your body is accustomed to your former food choices, but your sick cells will not be able to resist the high-quality nutrition you are feeding them on the detox. This is a period of adjustment. Good symptoms will kick in soon.

You may experience emotional and spiritual disruptions as well as physical symptoms. If you rely on junk food to quiet your negative emotions, all sorts of feelings and issues can surface when you stop, because you are not stuffing down your troubles with junk food. Your cells hold memories and the biochemistry of your unexpressed thoughts and feelings. Your emotional baggage is locked up in your cells. Those negative emotions are released along with chemical toxins. You might feel varying degrees of anger, anxiety, panic, depression, irritability, and hopelessness. When you detox, these feelings come to the surface. You are cleansing more than your body. Your thoughts, emotions, and spirit are also involved. You cannot have a healthy body, a healthy mind, and a healthy spirit if any of those aspects of yourself is out of sync.

> I started this detox because of thyroid issues, but it has also cleansed my spirit. During my healing crisis, I got out a lot of anger and negative emotions, and now I am left with energy and joy!
>
> T.F.

If you do not face the emotions that emerge and deal with them during your healing crisis, you will not be able to sustain the changes you are making in your body. You will fall back into your old eating habits. Very few people eat because they are hungry. They are eating because they are trying to fill an emotional hole or make themselves feel better. Food becomes comfort for whatever pain they are going through or have experienced. Your emotions will subside if you acknowledge them. As they do, your desire to eat will diminish.

One way to deal with your emotions is to express what you are feeling. Writing in your journal about your healing crisis is an effective way to engage those emotions. Putting what you are feeling into words has the power to diffuse them. What you have to do is allow yourself to observe the feelings that are emerging and to experience them. Doing so will give you great insight into what you are holding inside yourself. These negative thoughts and emotions are poisoning you just as much as toxic chemicals. Many detoxers turn to the community and describe what they are going through on our website, on Facebook, and on Twitter. You will get a lot of support from detoxers who have already been through what you are experiencing.

Be honest with the people around you about what is happening. It is a good idea to inform

> My wife and I are done with Day 7 now and feel we can make it. This really is a life-changing—well, "changing" is not quite the word—a catalytic life experience is more like it. We have had several eye-opening moments almost daily about all sorts of things that have been challenges for years! Somehow, now they come into perspective.
>
> T.R.

> Another major thing that helped me to stick to the program was the Facebook page. I checked the Facebook page daily, posted at least a couple of times a day, and made an effort to interact with other detoxers. This helped me stay motivated and accountable, because I could see other successful detoxers. It also helped me keep variety in my diet.
>
> I also tried just to focus on the here and now. I tried to take things hour by hour and not get caught up in any long-term weight-loss goals.
>
> Amy Guerich

those close to you that you might be in meltdown mode for a few days. You probably do not want to burst into tears at the office or bite your partner's head off. You can go off and sob or scream in privacy someplace. Or you can make a joke about it. Laughter always helps.

If you have had traumatic experiences, have been the victim of rape or physical abuse, or have had psychological problems in the past, you should consider whether you have healed emotionally. Any emotions you have suppressed could surface during this period. If you have unresolved issues and a troubled past, we recommend that you plan to see a therapist while you detox.

You will gradually become calmer, happier, and more vibrant as the days of your detox go by.

> You have to be committed because when you get headaches or feel nauseated or have body aches from detoxing, you have to be able to be mentally strong enough not to cave. Those brownies, etc. will be there any time of year, but carve out this time for you and do the detox and the transition right. Otherwise, you'll just chalk it up as something else you have tried that did not work. I'm proof it works. It was tough for me to lose weight, and I lost twenty-two pounds the first time I ever did the detox. I felt amazing. You owe this to yourself. Put your health first and you will succeed. You'll be so amazed that you'll wonder what took you so long to do it.
>
> Kimberly Kirkland Absher

Some detoxers become positively ecstatic, amazed by how centered, upbeat, and energized they feel. If you run into friends who have not seen you for a while, they will tell you how great you look and ask what you have done. They do not realize how beautiful health is.

We have some great techniques for minimizing the immediate effect that the release of toxins can have on your body and soul. These techniques are quick fixes that will buoy you up by helping your body eliminate the toxins being released. You can pick and choose from these suggested therapies to support and supplement your detox so that you can quickly pass through the crisis and feel the benefits of the detox. Make sure you continue to drink six to eight glasses of distilled water each day. If you feel particularly uncomfortable, you might consider doing a kidney flush or coffee enema, or getting a colonic. These treatments are described in the pages that follow.

EXTRA CREDIT

Just as extra credit gave you a chance to improve your grades at school, there are several things you can do to help move those toxins out of your body more quickly. These treatments focus on your organs of elimination. First, we will cover the treatments you can do yourself at home.

Detoxifying Bath

You remember that your skin is your largest organ of elimination. Taking a detoxifying bath once a week will stimulate the process. Just add the following ingredients to hot bathwater:

> **2 cups baking soda**, to neutralize acids
>
> **2 cups Epsom salts**, to give the water a higher ion content than the body to draw fluids from the body and toxins with them. Do not use Epsom salts if you have a rash or open wounds, because the salts will sting.
>
> **1 to 2 cups powdered oatmeal**, to act as an emollient to soothe dry skin problems. Put oatmeal in a blender or food processor and blend until it is the consistency of a fine powder.
>
> **A few drops of your favorite essential oils**, for their therapeutic properties

Just soaking in a bath once a week can support your detox. Soak for an hour. Continue to drink distilled water while in the bath. You probably do not need to be persuaded that taking a bath is therapeutic. What could be better after a long day?

Some Essential Oils and Their Emotional Healing Properties

Aromatherapy can help lift your spirits, soothe you, give you energy and focus, and relieve stress. Here are a few essences with their therapeutic properties.

Bergamot	Anger, anxiety, confidence, depression, stress, fatigue, fear, peace, happiness, insecurity, and loneliness
Chamomile	Anger, anxiety, depression, fear, irritability, loneliness, insomnia, stress
Eucalyptus	Concentration and memory
Grapefruit	Confidence, fear, depression, stress, happiness, and peace
Jasmine	Fatigue, exhaustion, burnout, stress, confidence, anger
Lavender	Anxiety, depression, irritability, panic attacks, stress
Lemon	Memory and concentration, fear, happiness, and peace
Patchouli	Fatigue and exhaustion, stress, frigidity
Peppermint	Concentration and memory, fatigue, exhaustion, burnout
Rose	Anger, anxiety, depression, grief, menopause, happiness and peace, loneliness, panic attacks, stress
Rosemary	Fatigue, exhaustion, burnout, confidence, concentration and memory
Sandalwood	Fear, grief, irritability, stress, depression, mental fatigue
Spearmint	Depression, mental fatigue
Vetiver	Anger, anxiety, exhaustion, insomnia, fear, grief, insecurity, stress
Ylang-ylang	Anger, depression, mood swings, PMS, stress

Most health food stores have a selection of essential oils. Whole Foods Market carries them in its beauty and bath departments. The Body Shop and Bath & Body Works make their own blends with different properties.

Dry Skin Brush

Brushing your skin with a natural bristle brush will slough off the dead cells on the outer layer, allowing your skin to breathe and to eliminate toxins. The most effective way to exfoliate the dead cells is to brush your skin when it is dry.

Use a brush made of vegetable fiber, with a long handle to help you reach everywhere. It will take about fifteen minutes to brush your entire body. The motion is up from your feet and hands and down on your torso from your shoulders. The movement is toward your heart.

1. Start at one of your feet and brush up the front of your leg to your waist in a circular motion with long strokes.
2. Repeat with the front of the other leg.
3. Do the same for the back of your legs to your waist.
4. Brush each arm up from your hands.
5. Brush down from your shoulders to your heart in front.
6. Brush up to your heart in front.
7. Brush up from your waist in back.

Brush hard enough to make your skin feel warm and become rosy, indicating that the top layers are sloughing off. Take a hot shower to relax and open your pores to let those toxins out. Cool down the water to close your pores as you do when you wash your face. This treatment is good for the detox, and great for your skin at any time.

Exercise

We do not advise doing an intense workout, a long run, an uphill bike ride, or a Zumba class while you are detoxing. It is not a good idea to stress your body to produce that high level of energy. You want to devote your energy to healing. That is not to say you should become a couch potato. Try to walk thirty minutes a day in the fresh air. Gentle yoga and meditation are good options.

At the retreat we use a rebounder, a small trampoline. Bouncing gently on a rebounder is one of the best exercises for detoxing. Some people do not have the energy to use a rebounder while detoxing. The movement stimulates and detoxes your lymphatic system. Jumping on a rebounder is often called "cellular exercise." It improves the flow of fluid between the cells. As you jump, the lymphatic system is mobilized, and toxins are expelled, causing weight loss. Rebounding helps to circulate oxygen in the body, stimulates metabolism, enhances digestion, and strengthens the immune system. Limit your rebounder use to ten minutes. Begin by bouncing every day for five to ten minutes twice a day. This can replace your daily walk. This exercise is great to incorporate into your post-detox routine.

Colon Cleanse

Clearing waste from your colon is an important aspect of good health. The standard American diet causes waste and synthetic substances to build up along the inside of the colon, creating a thick, slimy, black sludge. Toxins, additives, insufficient fiber, and low levels of digestive flora (good bacteria) or of enzymes contribute to the problem. Over time, the sludge hardens and develops the consistency of a rubber tire. Since the colon's inner walls are now covered with this sludge, the colon becomes desensitized; it does not feel the arriving waste material, and peristalsis is sluggish. Fecal matter stays in the colon longer and creates even more slime. Many people have between ten and twenty-five pounds of toxic fecal matter sitting in their colon.

When waste stays too long in your body, it rots, turns rancid, and smells. If you are not having one bowel movement a day, your body eventually protests and you experience at least one of these symptoms:

Excess abdominal weight—many people's bellies are stuffed
   with backed-up feces
Abdominal bloating and gas—these occur when decaying
   foods ferment

Acid reflux—when there is no room for food to go down,
it comes back up

Nausea or upset stomach—fermenting, rotting, rancid,
partially digested food can make you feel ill

Stomachaches—if you are not eliminating waste, your
entire digestive system expands to hold the waste and
pockets of gas

Body odor—sometimes the digestive system is so backed
up that the odor is excreted though the pores

Cleaning your colon is essential when you are detoxing. At the retreat, detoxers have a colonic each week. We describe the process in the Health Spa Therapies section on page 151. If you can go for a professional treatment, having a colonic is the one you should choose. Cleaning your colon will speed the detox process.

A symptom of your healing crisis might be constipation. Traditional medicine would use laxatives, primarily stool softeners and stimulants, to correct the problem. This is not a good idea. You should use laxatives very rarely, and not while you are detoxing. Laxatives are stimulants and add more toxins to your bloodstream. They can irritate the colon and make it spasm to purge some of its contents. Regular laxative use can damage the colon. Laxatives are habit forming. People rely on them so heavily that the laxatives make the colon sluggish. Once the habit is formed, bowels do not move without laxatives. Laxatives might help remove waste from the colon, but they do not touch the fecal matter that lines your intestinal walls.

You can make colon-cleansing teas and juices at home. While you are detoxing, the following tea is on the program:

LAXATIVE TEA

4 cups

⅛ teaspoon crushed dried licorice root inner bark
⅛ teaspoon flaxseeds, crushed
⅛ teaspoon dried senna leaf
1 quart distilled water
⅛ teaspoon carob pod seeds, crushed to powder
Stevia

Put the licorice root, flaxseeds, and senna in a tea ball. Bring the water to a boil in a pot over high heat. Add the tea ball and steep for 5 to 15 minutes, depending on how strong you want your tea. Add the carob powder and sweeten to taste.

Liver Cleanse

Your liver is so vital to your health that you want to keep it clean, which is easy to do.

HERBAL TEAS

Drinking the right herbal teas will stimulate bile secretion, help the liver detoxify, and help your colon with movement or peristalsis. You must be careful and check with your wellness practitioner before using them. Herbs are powerful. Teas are synergistically put together for you, so it is best to buy them in tea bags rather than putting them together yourself. These are some of the ingredients you should look for in a detox tea:

Barberry root bark
Orange grape root
Beet leaf
Burdock leaf and root
Dandelion leaf and root

Milk thistle
Red clover
Senna leaf
Aloe vera
Fennel seed
Licorice
Fenugreek
Yellow dock powder

These herbs might seem hard to get, but you would be surprised how easy they are to find. If you want to stick with ingredients you are more likely to have in your kitchen, here is an herbal liver detox you can make yourself.

HERBAL LIVER DETOX

3 servings

2 tablespoons dried milk thistle, chopped, or 2 tea bags
2 teaspoons dried rosemary leaves, chopped
2 teaspoons dried basil
⅛ teaspoon ground turmeric
Pinch of cayenne pepper
A few cilantro sprigs
1 quart distilled water
Stevia

1. Combine the milk thistle, rosemary, basil, turmeric, cayenne, and cilantro in a heatproof glass measuring cup or pitcher. Do not use a metal container.

2. Bring the water to a boil. Pour over the herbs and steep for 15 minutes.

3. Strain the tea through a fine-mesh sieve into a glass jar with a cover. Add stevia to taste.

4. Sip it slowly throughout the day. It is very potent, so do not drink it all at once. Save the rest for the next two weeks in a glass jar with a cover.

Coffee Enema

You might be squeamish when you see the word "enema," but if you give it a try, the results will surprise you. A coffee enema does more than just clean out your colon. The caffeine in coffee opens up the bile ducts, stimulating the liver to release fat-emulsifying bile. Caffeine also stimulates the liver to produce glutathione, an anti-oxidant that cleans your bloodstream. As we age and our toxic load increases, the liver produces less glutathione. By increasing your glutathione level, you boost your metabolism.

During the detox you should have a coffee enema once a week. Many detoxers make it a practice to have coffee enemas regularly.

You should use organic coffee for the cleanse. At the Martha's Vineyard Holistic Retreat, we use a disposable medical enema bag. We are not talking about the old-fashioned red rubber enema bag. Fleet makes a disposable one you can get at most drugstores and hospital supply stores, or order online. As long as you rinse the bag well with alcohol after using it, you can use it several times.

Most people like to do their enemas first thing in the morning, before showering. To prepare the solution:

1. Boil 6 to 8 tablespoons of organic ground coffee in 6 cups distilled water for at least 5 minutes but no more than 15 minutes. If you are sensitive to caffeine, use 4 to 6 tablespoons.
2. Allow the coffee to cool until it feels barely warm when you put a few drops on the inside of your wrist, as you would test a baby's bottle. You might want to prepare the coffee the night before your enema and reheat it for a minute to warm it up.

3. Carefully strain the coffee to remove all the grounds. Grounds can clog up the tubing of the enema bag.
4. Pour the solution into the enema bag, making sure the tube is clamped. Take the bag to your bathroom. Hang the bag approximately 4 feet above your head, if you were lying down. The height determines how fast the coffee will flow. A towel rack is usually a good height.
5. Place a waterproof "blue" pad covered by a dark-colored towel on the floor of the bathroom.
6. Lubricate the applicator tip with olive oil, vitamin E oil, virgin coconut oil, or KY Jelly.
7. Lie down on your right side and insert the tip of the tube into your rectum. Gently push about 6 inches of the tube into your rectum.
8. Release the clamp and let the coffee slowly flow into your rectum. Count slowly to five and then clamp the tube. You want to let in a half-cup of solution at a time. Repeat until all the solution is used. You do not have to clamp the tube if you are feeling comfortable with the flow.
9. Try to retain the coffee for at least 10 or up to 15 minutes. If you hold the coffee too long, you may absorb the caffeine, which might make you wired and jittery. If you feel a mild cramp, let a little of the coffee out. It might be gas.
10. If you feel a hard cramp, head to the toilet. Place your feet on a low stool.
11. Push the feces and coffee out. Normally you should not push when you are having a bowel movement. Pushing during a coffee enema opens your gallbladder, cleansing your liver and bile ducts.

Most detoxers feel fabulous after a coffee enema. They say they feel lighter, exuberant, and cleaner. So get over your reservations and just do it.

For extra credit, the exercise, detoxifying bath, and lymphatic body brushing should be easy to incorporate into your detox. The specific cleanses are not that challenging. You can use them to replace a cup of tea. You may be resistant to the idea of a coffee enema, but it is well worth overcoming your aversion. Some detoxers have become addicted to the treatment because it makes them feel so good. You can do all of these treatments at home with very little expense. If you want to re-create the retreat experience, there are professional treatment options that support the detox as well.

HEALTH SPA THERAPIES

If you were at the Martha's Vineyard Holistic Retreat, you would select a spa treatment a day. You can treat yourself to the therapies we offer at the retreat that support your detox. Here are a few therapies our detoxers find invaluable.

Infrared Sauna

If you have access to an infrared sauna, maybe at your gym or health club, you should use it once a week while you are on the detox. Sweating is good for eliminating toxins. Saunas help the body to rid itself of heavy metals like lead, mercury, and nickel. Saunas help you to lose weight by increasing your metabolism. The heat increases the flexibility of your muscles and joints. If you do not have access to a sauna, you might be able to get a day pass at another gym or a YMCA/YWCA. Some Y's now have infrared saunas.

Colonics

Colon hydrotherapy is a way of cleansing the colon, and you already know how important that is. This therapy must be administered by a trained colon hydrotherapist with professional equipment. Colonics have deeper cleaning power than enemas. The colon is roughly five and a half to six feet long and can stretch to two and a half to three inches in diameter. Colonics use multiple infusions of water; an enema uses only one infusion. The water in an enema bag is sufficient to stimulate peristalsis only in the lower one-third of your colon. Peristalsis is the constriction and relaxation of muscles in your intestine. The wavelike movement pushes waste from your colon. Colonics cleanse the entire length of the colon.

The reason to have a colonic is that fecal matter can accumulate and harden in the colon. The buildup of fecal matter can:

- Lead to constipation
- Interfere with the absorption of water and nutrients
- Allow harmful colon bacteria and yeast to grow
- Cause stagnant toxins to be absorbed into the bloodstream through the wall of the colon

When you have a closed-system colonic, the colon therapist gently inserts the base of a Y-shaped speculum about an inch or two into your rectum. The hose attached to the narrow side of the Y directs a stream of purified water into the colon from the hydrotherapy unit. Fecal material is eliminated through the other hose and empties into a closed waste system. The water causes the muscles of the colon to contract and push the waste into the tube. When your bowels move, there are no sounds, smells, spills, or mess. During the colonic, the therapist might massage your abdomen lightly to loosen impacted waste material and to facilitate elimination.

As the fecal matter is eliminated, it flows past a window in the colonic machine, which provides a view of how well your digestive system is working. The therapist can observe whether you are chewing your food well enough; if stool has become impacted in your colon; whether *Candida* or yeast is overgrown; and if you have excess mucus, bacteria, toxins, or parasites. The process is very revealing about the state of your body.

The colon is rinsed and cleansed several times during the process. After the colonic, the therapist leaves the room, and you sit on a toilet to pass any residual water and stool.

The average person needs three or four sessions to clean out the entire colon. When you have a colonic, you will feel cleaner, lighter, and more energetic right away. After a colonic, you have a visceral sense of how toxins weigh you down.

There have been advances in colon hydrotherapy. With an open-system colonic, you eliminate into a basin or channel that leads to the toilet. The speculum is much smaller than the one used in closed systems. The flow is very gentle and gravity-fed, so some people find it more comfortable. After initial guidance, you help the therapist with the process by regulating the flow of water. With experience, you can do the colonic alone.

At the retreat, detoxers have a colonic each week. If your budget will allow, you should do the same. If you can afford only one colonic, schedule an appointment for the third day of your detox. The best way to find a colonic therapist is by referral. You can visit the website of the International Association for Colon Hydrotherapy (www.i-act.org) to make certain a therapist is certified.

Chi Machine

The chi machine helps to detox your body as you lie flat on your back with your ankles or calves resting on the machine. At the retreat, this is hands down the favorite form of exercise. The machine is designed to improve the movement of chi (life-force energy) in the body. The machine gently moves the body from side to side in a figure eight, the same way a goldfish swims. The movement is comparable to a masseuse holding your ankles and swinging you from side to side after a massage. The movement maximizes the body's natural absorption of oxygen. Oxygenation raises your metabolic rate, increases your energy and focus, and improves your blood circulation.

Aside from oxygenating your tissues, the movement stimulates the lymphatic system to move and to detox. The chi machine reduces muscle soreness, tension, and stiffness, reducing body aches and pains. The movement aligns the spine. It relaxes you, putting you in a meditative state of calmness. This movement is particularly helpful for detoxers who are significantly overweight or obese, older, or sedentary. A hour a day on the chi machine is very helpful. You will find chi machines at alternative healing centers.

Many detoxers, particularly those who find it difficult to exercise, buy their own chi machines. To find the machine we use at the retreat, check www.DrRoniChiMachine.com. You can also find a good chi machine by contacting Info@TheChiMachine.com. The toll-free number is 877-369-8305.

Lymph Drainage Massage

When you think of massage, you probably think of reducing muscular tension. A lymph drainage massage is a very light massage that encourages the flow of lymph in the body and drains the lymph nodes. As you remember, the lymphatic system needs motion to move lymph. This type of massage gets your lymph moving to carry away toxins. Other benefits include draining swollen tissue and supporting the immune system. You can see how a lymph drainage massage would contribute to your detox. Check day spas in your town. Some dermatologists have a massage therapist on the staff because lymph massage improves the skin's appearance.

Inch-Loss Body Wrap

Body wraps take off inches rather than pounds. You can concentrate on specific trouble spots like stomach, hips, or thighs. Wraps encourage elimination of toxins that cause you to bloat. Spas use special mixes of herbs and mineral salts that stimulate circulation and extract toxins.

If you feel bloated or flabby, an inch-loss body wrap will help firm you up. After a few treatments, the cellulite in your skin will start to smooth out. Doing a body wrap once a week during the detox can noticeably improve your appearance.

There is a homemade version you can try. We have to warn you that it is messy. You will need eight bath towels that you do not mind getting stained, a thermal blanket, a regular blanket, and a plastic sheet or drop cloth to wrap yourself in. Here are two solutions to apply to your skin. You can powder the herbs or sea vegetable in your food processor. The nourishment of the wrap will be absorbed through your skin.

AT-HOME BODY WRAP

Herbal Body Wrap
2 quarts distilled water
1 cup Epsom salts
1 cup powdered dried herbs, or 30 drops essential oils
     (lavender, chamomile, ginger, grapefruit, lemongrass, and
     clary sage are good choices, alone or in combination)
2 cups bentonite clay

Sea Vegetable Body Wrap
2 quarts distilled water
1 cup sea salt
1 cup powdered sea vegetable such as kelp or dulse
2 cups bentonite clay

TO MAKE THE WRAP SOLUTION:
Bring the water and salt to a boil in a very large stainless-steel pot. Turn off the heat and add the herbs or sea vegetable. Stir in with a wooden spoon. Add the clay and stir until it dissolves. Let cool for 10 to 15 minutes, until comfortable to the touch.

BODY WRAP METHOD:
   1. Create a place to lie down. The bottom layer should be a waterproof thermal blanket, the middle layer a normal blanket, the top layer a plastic sheet.

2. Play some music you find relaxing. Make sure you have a tall glass of water within reach. Staying hydrated is important.

3. Dry-brush your skin and then take a warm shower to open your pores.

4. Sit down on the layered blankets.

5. Dip the towels into the mix one at a time.

6. Starting at your ankles, wrap each leg with a lengthwise towel.

7. Wrap a towel around your stomach and another around your midriff.

8. Wrap your chest and shoulders.

9. Wrap each arm, lengthwise again.

10. Lie down and cocoon by wrapping the three layers of thermal blanket, regular blanket, and plastic sheet around you. Relax for 60 minutes.

11. Take a tepid bath after the body wrap and drink more water.

12. During this peaceful hour, the body wrap will draw excess fluid and toxins from your body. This will result in temporary weight loss and a loss of inches.

Cellulite Treatments

Few of us manage to avoid "orange peel syndrome" or "cottage cheese skin," also known as cellulite. The dimpled appearance of skin on the stomach and back and front of the thighs is caused by fat deposits just below the surface of the skin. Though genetics and hormones play a part, what you eat is a factor. If you eat foods filled with toxins, processed foods, salt, sugar, preservatives, fried foods, and alcohol, your body becomes overwhelmed and cannot eliminate efficiently. These substances build up in fat cells. Though cellulite creams are available, seeing a massage therapist will give you much better results.

Cellulite treatments begin with rubbing into the area a special cellulite cream that penetrates deeply into the skin, allowing nutrients to enter. The therapist uses special movements to help dissolve the lumps: percussion, vigorous palpation, circular movements, pressure, and stroking. The more skillful the therapist, the better the treatment works.

We use products made by Sybaritic at the retreat. Oxygen Botanicals Celliminate is its cellulite cream. It also makes a body contouring oil for inch loss and use in body wraps. Its phone number is 952-888-8282, and its address is 9220 James Avenue South, Minneapolis, MN 55431.

TROUBLESHOOTING YOUR HEALING

Even letter-perfect detoxers sometimes have difficulty dropping those pounds. Some lose inches but not as many pounds as they would like. Others plateau during the detox because the weight of the fat they are losing is offset by increasing muscle mass. Muscle tissue weighs more than fat. Though weight loss can be slower than normal for many reasons, people in this predicament often have similar symptoms. Detoxers report on a number of troubling symptoms during the detox, including

Bloating and gas after eating soup or drinking juice
Sugar and carbohydrate cravings
Irregularity
Fatigue or tiredness on waking
Feeling very hot or cold
Depression and anxiety

Experiencing new side effects from medication. Your cells are dumping residual medication into your bloodstream that can cause side effects you have never had before.

Bad breath

If you are stuck at the same weight or have any of these symptoms, here are some home remedies that may jump-start your weight loss and get you through your healing crisis. If these quick fixes do not work, you should check with your doctor to determine whether you have a thyroid problem or hormonal imbalance that needs attention.

Intestinal discomfort: Take extra enzymes or increase your daily aloe vera supplement.

Excessive cravings: Take Glucofast, a supplement that supports weight loss and healthy blood glucose levels. It is composed of natural botanicals, vitamins, and minerals. If you cannot find it in your health food store, you can order it online.

Constipation: See a colon therapist or increase your aloe vera gel to twice a day.

Fatigue: Add the sea vegetables kelp or dulse to your evening soup. They provide extra minerals, sodium, and iodine. If you feel most fatigued after exercise, you may need additional minerals.

Sluggish metabolism: Take Glucofast.

Depression: If you are taking an antidepressant, consult your doctor. If you are not, add essential fatty acids and protein drinks containing amino acids to the detox. This will help to relieve depression but may slow weight loss.

Extreme changes in body temperature: If you have hot flashes, feel cold all the time, or have cold hands and feet, ask your doctor to perform a hormone panel to evaluate your hormone levels. If you feel your menstrual cycle is interfering with weight loss, try progesterone cream, which helps with hot flashes as well. If you are cold all the time, consult your doctor about a thyroid panel.

Candida: Yeast imbalances can cause sugar or carbohydrate cravings. To discover if you have a problem, take a *Candida* test at an alternative practitioner's office. If you test positive, add protein shakes to your detox. Juices contain many complex carbohydrates that will feed the yeast or slow your weight loss.

Bad breath: Dieting often gives people bad breath. At the start of the detox that might happen, but as your digestive tract cleans out, the problem should correct itself. Until it does, chlorophyll has a deodorizing effect. If your breath is troubling you, have a shot of wheatgrass each day. Chlorophyll tablets are also available. Chewing fresh herbs will give you sweet breath. Mint, parsley, rosemary, sage, thyme, and wintergreen are the best for this purpose.

*   *   *

You are ready to start the first twenty-one days of the detox. This is one of the best gifts you could ever give yourself. Tomorrow will be the beginning of a new way of life for you. You have made a decision to change your relationship with food. Be prepared to feel better than you have in your entire life. The next thirty days will take you to a place of clarity, vitality, and lightness. Your skinny jeans will fit again, and you will glow with health. We almost wish we were in your shoes—ready to experience the detox for the first time—because it is so transformative and exciting. Enjoy every minute of it.

Detox Success Story

I DO NOT NEED MEDICATION
TO MAINTAIN A HEALTHY MIND

Before I started the detox program I was feeling heavy, and my mind was not clear. I had been in a bad car accident a month after I had gotten married to the man of my dreams . . .

I was in a lot of pain . . . and was becoming toxic to myself. I was taking medication for postpartum depression. Mind you, my daughter is now three years old. I am not a depressed person, but I had become dependent on this medication. For some reason, I thought I could not survive without it.

The Martha's Vineyard Diet Detox has helped me prove to myself I can do anything I put my mind to and that I am a strong individual. I do not need medication to maintain a healthy mind. I just need to take better care of myself. I have lost twenty-two pounds and need to lose only eight more to meet my personal goal . . . For the first time in three years, I am not taking medication, and I don't feel the need for it anymore.

Inspired by the Bible, I began to think of my body as a temple that I needed to take care of and cleanse, because it is a gift. That Bible verse helped me to pull through the healing crisis and the temptations . . . Keeping it free of toxins and negativity is my new goal.

R.G.

CHAPTER 9

MAKE A DAZZLING REENTRY: THE TRANSITION

You have done it! You have completed the first twenty-one days of the 1 Pound a Day Diet Detox. You are flying high. You have lost weight, and as the pounds melted off, it seemed effortless. Judging from what other detoxers report, we feel safe to assume that you have not felt this good in a very long time.

We encourage you to share your experiences and the results of the first twenty-one days on our website (www.mvdietdetox.com) or on Twitter or Facebook. You have followed a very structured program for three weeks and have achieved remarkable results. You have reduced your toxic load, and your body and cells are as clean as they have ever been and are wide open to absorb nutrients. The last thing you want to do is to pick up where you left off.

Your body will be very sensitive to the toxins in processed and junk food. On Day 22, you will not be "rewarding" yourself

> Well, today is Day 21 and I feel fantastic! This is the second detox I have completed for a total weight loss of thirty-two pounds! I am the same weight I was in college. I have so much energy I've rejoined my local dojo, and I'm back to training. My BMI has dropped by 2.2. I'm feeling fantastic. I can see my abs again—which I'm pretty stoked about! I think people are going to think I have shares in the book or something.
>
> S.H.
> ～

with toxic treats and foods you have done without. If you do, your body will react. You might have an energy crash, or get bloated, or develop a rash, or get sick to your stomach. Returning suddenly to toxic eating habits will disrupt your smooth-running metabolism and cause you to gain weight immediately. Listen to your body. It will be communicating with you about what foods you should stay away from. Your fresh new cells will be experiencing these toxins for the first time. You will feel the shock in your body as it reacts to toxic foods. Making the transition to healthy eating will be easier, because your body will let you know when the foods you eat are hurting it.

Warning: Do not consume cigarettes, alcoholic beverages, or illegal drugs for eleven days after the detox. As a general rule, avoid highly toxic substances for half the number of days you have detoxed. This rule will come into play if you do the tune-up detoxes covered in Chapter 14.

Do not let our first book, *21 Pounds in 21 Days*, mislead you. The detox is not over in twenty-one days. The process is thirty days long. The last nine days of the detox are designed to help you transition to eating solid food again. A controlled reentry is essential if you want to stabilize your weight loss and lock in the improvements you have seen in the past three weeks. During this nine-day period, the program gradually awakens your digestive system by reintroducing all of the food groups back to your diet.

I am going to eat lettuce tomorrow! I find it hard to believe that I would ever get so excited about eating lettuce. I've lost thirty-six pounds and feel terrific. Now I am focused on eating correctly (I've known how for a long time, but chose not to) and exercising (same). My mental clarity is phenomenal. These results are amazing. I may do the full detox later in the year.

Robert Cohen

You start with a salad and end with animal protein. During the nine-day transition, eat modest portions of food. Do not overeat. If you do, you will really feel it.

You are feeling great. Why ruin it? Eat more slowly than you usually do. Don't inhale your food. Take time to enjoy what you are eating. Try chewing each bite a hundred times. That will get digestion started in your mouth, making your digestive system work less.

Pay close attention to how your body reacts to what you are eating. From constipation to itchy skin, record your reactions in your journal. You might discover food intolerances you were never aware you had, because your body was so overloaded it was reacting to everything all the time.

We want your reentry to be safe. We do not want the transition to undo the good you have done for your body.

> Doing the transition after detoxing was not difficult. It was as if my body had taken charge. Many types of food I used to eat on a regular basis no longer seemed appealing to me. I was a steak person. Once I finished doing the detox, I had no desire to eat red meat.
>
> Jacqueline Malloy

NINE DAYS TO EASE BACK TO HEALTHY EATING

Breaking Your Detox, Day 22: Add 1 Portion Raw or Cooked Vegetables

Add 10 to 12 ounces of raw vegetable salad or cooked vegetables with no dressing, oil, or vinegar. You can use Bragg Liquid Aminos or fresh lemon juice to dress the vegetables or salad.

Breaking Your Detox, Day 23: Add Fresh Fruit

Add a bowl of cut-up berries to what you eat on Day 22. This must be eaten two hours before or after meals. The fruit could be a good midmorning or midafternoon snack.

Breaking Your Detox, Day 24: Add Whole Grains

Add one serving of a whole grain such as steel-cut oatmeal (not instant), brown rice, or quinoa. You might want to put some brown rice or barley in your soup or broth.

Breaking Your Detox, Day 25: Add Essential Fatty Acids

Two essential fatty acids, omega-3 and omega-6, cannot be synthesized in the body. These fatty acids affect the functioning of all tissues of the body. Deficiencies produce abnormalities in the liver and kidney, changes in blood, decreased immune function, depression, and dryness and scaliness of skin. The benefits of adequate intake of these fatty acids include prevention of atherosclerosis, reduced incidence of heart disease and stroke, and relief from colitis symptoms and menstrual and joint pain. Though there are food sources for omega-3 and omega-6 fatty acids (see page 194), you can take an essential fatty acid liquid or capsule, or flaxseed oil, which you can buy at your local health food store.

Breaking Your Detox, Day 26: Add Protein Shakes

Even though there is protein in whole grains, which you had on Day 24, you may be craving protein. Protein is an important component of every cell in the body. Take away the water and about 75 percent of your remaining weight is protein, an important component of every cell in your body. Your hair and nails are mostly made of protein. Your body uses protein to build and repair tissues. Proteins function as building blocks for bones, muscles, cartilage, skin, and blood. Your body uses protein to make enzymes, which power many chemical reactions, and hormones, the body's messengers. Our recipes for protein shakes begin on page 237.

> Just finished my detox, and I can honestly say I have never felt better! I am down to 119 pounds from 131 pounds. As I introduce foods back into my system, I am much more able to gauge what my body can and cannot tolerate. For years, I have eaten various foods and not considered the effects they were having on my body. From completing the detox, I was able to learn what my body likes and doesn't like and can continue to feel great because of it.
>
> Alisha Walker

Breaking Your Detox, Day 27: Add Whole Food Sources of Protein

Add a portion of eggs, soy, nuts, or legumes and beans such as pinto beans, black-eyed peas, kidney beans, and lentils. You can put a hard-boiled egg on your salad or enjoy ¼ cup of nuts.

At this point you will stop eating soup at night.

Breaking Your Detox, Day 28: Add White Meat

Add 3 to 4 ounces of boiled, broiled, or baked fish or skinless chicken to your diet. The serving size should be about the size of a deck of cards. The fish should be wild, not farm-raised. The chicken should be free range and should not contain hormones or antibiotics. In general, try not to consume animal muscle protein more than three times a week. That means you should not eat chicken or fish one day in the remaining transition days. Try rice and beans instead.

> Just finished the detox—the best New Year present I ever gave myself. This is not the end. It is truly the beginning of a new way of life.
>
> C.M.

Breaking Your Detox, Day 29: Add Red Meat (Optional)

If you chose to eat red meat, you can add 3 to 4 ounces on Day 29.

Begin Dr. Roni's Healthy Eating Plan on Day 30

This is your first day on Doctor Roni's Healthy Eating Plan. You will be eating every two to three hours, taking enzymes when you have a meal that involves chewing, and continuing to drink water on odd hours. Part 3 of the book gives you a blueprint for eating well for the rest of your life. You will find how your daily nourishment will be structured on page 232.

Detox Success Story
SPOTLIGHT ON FOOD SENSITIVITIES

The idea to do a detox program was attractive at first because it was a new concept for me, and I was curious to see if I could accomplish and complete the program. Not only was I interested in dropping a few pounds, but also, above all, I wanted to see what foods agreed or disagreed with me once the "reintroduction" process was to begin.

On the program, each day's success strengthened my self-esteem and got me in gear for the new day. I was feeling pretty good quickly—just a little tired at first. Feeling great came at about Week 2. I became brighter, fresher, ready to go. I saw the pounds dropping, but I was most interested to see if my allergies, breathing, and rash were food related.

I had been to a dermatologist, a GI specialist, and an infectious disease MD as well. No one could tell me what was going on with my arms. I had a rash that looked like infectious dermatitis that had been spreading. It was awful looking and itched like crazy. I would wake up in the morning with blood on the sheets. I must have been scratching during my sleep. It was horrible. I was given creams, ointments, pills, soaks, and other remedies. Nothing helped.

My sprits skyrocketed once I saw that my arms were clearing up! Eureka! I thought. Had I found the cure? If not, then maybe I had at least found the cause of the rash.

Initially, the most important part of this program for me was the transition from detoxing, the reintroduction of foods. I was able to monitor and see firsthand which foods triggered poor reactions in my body. This was a very deliberate time for me. I was keeping a list of my food, quantity, and reactions observed and felt. I found that gluten plays an important part in my life. I react fast and severely to it. Learning to try to eliminate it from my diet has been a new standard for me.

Once I tried breads and cakes, my arms went right back into rash mode! Nasty! I still love a bite or two of a baked goodie, but I know the consequences, and I also know that I have the tools to control outbreaks. I repeat the detox whenever I need a physical or mental lift. Not only does it lighten the scale, but it also reminds me that I can see personal success on a daily basis if I stay focused.

Renée Convers

PART 3

~

KEEP IT
GOING

CHAPTER 10

STAY LIGHT

You have done it! You have finished the 1 Pound a Day Diet Detox. You look and feel better than you have in years. You never want to feel the way you used to again. You are ready to give your fat clothes away, because you are not going back there. You can see and feel how much lighter you are without those toxins clogging up your body and weighing you down. You are a living example of what eating clean does for you. You are ready to make a commitment to change the way you nourish your body forever. Keep It Going, the last part of the book, will help you make that change with Dr. Roni's Healthy Eating Plan, a program for the right way to eat for the rest of your life.

Dr. Roni's plan will intro-

I finished my detox three weeks ago, and I just want to say you can keep the weight off. I lost fifteen pounds and I have not gained any of it back. My scale goes up and down by one pound here and there. I attribute it to water weight and sodium intake. Even though I haven't lost any more weight, I am still losing inches. I am exercising much more now than during the detox, and I can see my body toning up. I am eating completely clean, and about 60 to 75 percent raw. Also, I use Monday as a cleansing day and only drink fresh juice and a raw nut milk that day. I plan to do a tune-up every three months.

T.M.

❧

duce you to a way of eating that will make yo-yo dieting a thing of the past. In the chapters that follow, we will show you how to keep off the weight you lost, supercharge your energy, and maintain good health for life. Dr. Roni's Healthy Eating Plan maximizes cellular nourishment and creates a biochemical environment in which metabolism stabilizes, weight loss becomes permanent, and healing takes place naturally. In this section of the book, you will learn:

- Five Principles of Healthy Eating that you can apply to any dietary philosophy—omnivore, carnivore, piscatarian, vegetarian, or vegan
- Self-defense strategies to protect your body from the conditions and chronic diseases that inevitably occur as a result of eating the highly processed foods at the heart of the standard American diet (SAD)
- How to increase your energy level, lose excess pounds, and stabilize your weight by eating foods in metabolically correct combinations
- How to maximize the antiaging properties inherent in certain foods to remove years from your face and body
- What you need to know to reset your metabolism so that you stop gaining weight
- Techniques to help stabilize your blood sugar and stave off food binges and cravings that jeopardize your weight and health
- Ways to keep your internal body chemistry in a state in which the cells detoxify themselves
- How changing your food choices can eliminate fuzzy thinking and indecisiveness while increasing your ability to focus
- Why it is important to build at least an annual detox into your lifestyle

DO NOT BE UNDERMINED

You have to be prepared for some surprising reactions to what you have accomplished. Not everyone will react with enthusiasm to the way you have changed. Your "frenemies" will put you down, saying things like "Don't lose more weight, you're going to be skin and bones," or "Losing weight so fast isn't good for you," or "Of course, you lost weight, you stopped eating. You're going to blow up now that you can eat again. Starvation diets don't work." Do not let these people get to you. They do not know what they are talking about. Most likely, they are envious. They would love to be in your shoes. You have to learn to shrug off their comments. Knowing that you look so good that some colleagues, friends, and family feel the need to knock you down should be a consolation. You have set yourself apart. You can be confident that you are an example of what eating well can do for you. Who knows? When they see you are unflappable, you might inspire these people to try the 1 Pound a Day Diet Detox themselves.

Even worse than their comments, jealous people will try to entice you to eat badly. "Well, that's over," they might say. "Let's go celebrate at an all-you-can-eat buffet." You might want to join them, but just eat right wherever you go. We will give you advice later in this chapter about how to order in restaurants. Do not fall back into your old eating habits. It is strange to imagine that seeing you regress will please some people, but that is human nature. People are competitive and do not want others to do better than themselves. Some would rather be negative and deny how great you look than put themselves on the right track.

If these unkind reactions bother you, you can describe the situations on our Twitter and Facebook pages, which you can reach through our website, www.mvdietdetox.com. There are plenty of detoxers who have experienced the same negativity. They will be there to support you, to let you know that you are not alone. They will probably share some great zinger comebacks. You will have an easier time keeping off the weight you have lost if you tap into the community ready to support you. If you feel your resolve wavering, check in with people who have been there. Fellow detoxers will be quick to let you know that no one is perfect. Their stories will help you to stay on track.

THE 75/25 PERCENT SOLUTION

You may be thinking right now, "You mean I can never have fried chicken, a cheeseburger, or gooey cheese on a slice of French bread again?" Don't worry—Dr. Roni has a 75/25 percent solution. When it comes to changing the way you eat, we expect progress, not perfection. If you eat on the plan 75 percent of the time, you will be taking a dramatic step forward and will do just fine. You will improve that split over time, because you will become aware of how much better you look and feel when you live by the rules. Eventually you will be eating well 80 percent of the time, and then 90 percent.

> I have lost twenty-two pounds, and I'm still going to continue to eat, exercise, and plan for a healthier lifestyle. The detox has been a great journey for me to learn more about myself . . . Forgiveness is the key when faltering—pace yourself, comfort and peace will come. Take care and love yourself.
>
> Phyllis Jennings

People approach this 75/25 split in various ways. James eats very carefully until he travels, but then he eats whatever he wants. He goes for five months following the rules, then he has a week or two of not paying close attention. Some detoxers blow out at holidays and parties and eat carefully the rest of the time. If you look at the calendar, you will find at least one holiday a month. Others like to have a cheat day on Sunday, when they eat whatever they want. You will find a pattern that works for you.

You might indulge in a giant burger and supersize fries, but the memory of the bloated feeling and indigestion that followed will make you think twice the next time you find yourself at a fast-food restaurant. Remember, your body has become sensitized to toxins, additives, and foods that weigh you down. James was at a formal dinner in London recently. He could not resist the elaborate beef dish and the sweet desserts that were served to him, and he paid for it. After coming off a seven-day detox, he should have known better. He woke up the next day with horrible blisters on his lips. We are not saying you should not eat beef, but in this instance, it was clear that James's body reacted to what he ate. You have to respond to the signs your body sends you. When the body is in a clean state with less acidity, you tend to have a healing crisis when you go fast-forward into antibiotic-, hormone-, and additive-filled food. That is why James crashed into a bad state.

The worst thing you can do is to cheat just a little bit each day. This stresses the immune system and raises blood sugar and insulin levels, canceling out the good work of the entire day. Daily cheating—say, a couple of cookies each day or a glass or two of red wine after work—can make you feel hungry, tired, and maybe even depressed. A blood sugar swing during the evening may disrupt your sleep and make you feel tired the next day. Instead of cheating a little every day, give yourself permission to take an occasional break from Dr. Roni's Healthy Eating Plan now and then.

If you are going to cheat, you might as well enjoy yourself. You are allowed to have a blowout once in a while. Dr. Roni believes that it is fine to take off every now and then. Do not feel like a failure if you do. Just get right back on Dr. Roni's Healthy Eating Plan. You will continue to improve and increase your healing.

You do not have to become a total ascetic to keep the weight off. You just have to know how to handle those times that you stray. If you lose it for a while, you can do a one-day, weekend, or seven-day detox by following the schedules outlined in Chapter 14, Your Body Deserves a Five-Star Vacation and Regular Getaways.

THE FIVE PRINCIPLES OF HEALTHY EATING

For almost twenty years, Dr. Roni has taught her principles of healthy eating at the Martha's Vineyard Holistic Retreat. When people come to the retreat or consult with Dr. Roni, they are usually confused and overwhelmed. Should they eat this food or that one? One week, a study says that coffee, chocolate, eggs—whatever the food of the day may be—is good for you. The next week studies show that same food is a threat to your health, causing heart disease, cancer, or another serious ailment. From low-calorie cookies to fat-free salad dressings to low-fat ice cream, you can count on manufacturers to slap a health label on any processed food they think can make them some money. Sifting through all the conflicting information to figure out what is right for you can be overwhelming.

Dr. Roni's five simple principles will set you straight. These basic rules hold the key to shedding excess weight, maintaining that weight loss, and improving your health. These principles apply no matter what you like to eat—whether you love sinking your teeth into a nice juicy steak from time to time, eat only fish or fowl, or are a committed vegetarian. It does not matter whether you shop at Whole Foods Market or Walmart. These guidelines help align your organs and optimize your metabolism so that everything is working together toward a common goal: digesting your food efficiently and effectively so that you have energy and your body heals and regenerates itself. The five principles form the foundation of a lifestyle change that will carry on the good work you have done on the 1 Pound a Day Diet Detox. We have covered a couple of the principles earlier in the book but will tailor our discussion to apply post-detox. Here are the rules to live by.

1. **Consume maximum nutrition in small doses every few hours.** You will be continuing a scaled-down version of the schedule you followed during the detox in your everyday life. Instead of eating three square meals a day and a snack, you will eat small, densely nutritious

doses of food every few hours. The schedule appears later in this chapter on page 176. It is important to continue to nourish your body with antioxidants, live juices, greens, and enzymes for maximum nutrition. Eating this way keeps your blood sugar levels even, increases your energy, prevents cravings, reduces the calories the body stores as fat, and prevents digestive disturbances like indigestion, bloating, and gas.

2. **Minimize toxic ingredients.** Your food consumption on the detox was very limited. Now that you are facing the whole world of food, you have to make informed choices to eat clean and green. Whether BPA that leaches out of cans and plastics or artificial flavors, coloring, or preservatives found in processed foods, toxins damage your organs, cloud your thinking, and disrupt your body's balance, making it store more fat and causing disease.

3. **Eat high-alkaline, high-fiber foods.** Eating foods that reduce the acidity of your body will keep you healthy. When the fluids in your body are excessively acidic, every part of your body is weakened, and this condition can lead to serious liver, kidney, and heart problems. When your acid/alkaline balance leans toward acid, it can cause weight gain, an increase in blood pressure, premature aging, and diabetes. Chapter 12 will show you how to regain a healthy balance in your body. Eating high-fiber foods, as you have learned earlier, can reduce cravings, correct blood-sugar swings, minimize digestive problems, and keep the body from accumulating fat.

4. **Combine foods in ways that are metabolically correct.** When you eat foods in combinations that optimize metabolism, you keep your body systems from competing with each other and causing digestive problems, low energy, weight gain, and inflammation. Chapter 13 will give you guidelines.

5. **Detoxify regularly.** You may not be able to do much about many of the environmental, chemical, and food toxins you are exposed to, but you can act to reduce your toxic load. You can make detoxing a regular part of your self-care regimen. Whether you choose a quick weekend or seven-day detox or the full 1 Pound a Day Diet Detox, you have to give your body a chance to rest and recuperate. Chapter 14 will cover the need to rid your body of noxious chemicals on a regular basis.

In this part of the book you will learn how to make these rules so much a part of your life that they become automatic—like brushing your teeth in the morning. We will share practical advice on how to deal with the challenges of eating well in an unhealthy world.

ADJUSTING YOUR MEAL TIMING

With Dr. Roni's Healthy Eating Plan, you will be nourishing your body at regular intervals during the day with a schedule similar to the one you followed on the detox. You will continue to have the berry antioxidant drink or powder, the green juice powder, the enzyme pills, and the aloe vera as part of your regular routine. This will deliver high-density nutrients to your body at regular intervals and will stabilize your blood sugar levels. Here is a schedule of food and nutritional drinks you should consume each day:

DR. RONI'S HEALTHY EATING PLAN

Wake-Up: High-density antioxidant berry drink
Breakfast: Protein smoothie or protein breakfast
Snack: Fresh vegetable juice or green juice powder drink
Lunch: Enzymes
    Vegetables and/or complex carbohydrates*

Snack: Healthy snack—see list on page 197

Dinner: Enzymes

    Protein with veggies, or soup meal

Bedtime: Aloe

*Complex carbohydrates are "good carbohydrates" like whole grains, fruits, and vegetables. Simple carbohydrates, such as products made with white flour and sweets, break down into glucose very quickly and cause a spike in blood sugar. Complex carbohydrates take longer to break down in your body, producing sustained energy.

Do not forget to stay hydrated. You should consume at least eight glasses of beverage a day. For every pound you weigh, you need one-half ounce of fluid intake a day. If you weigh 150 pounds, you should drink 75 ounces of fluid, or a little more than nine cups. This figure varies depending on how much exercise you do. For a precise measurement, there are many calculators available online. You can find one on the BrainMeasures.com website. If you have trouble re-membering to drink your water, try drinking a glass on the odd hours of the day.

This schedule describes your new daily food routine in general terms. The chapters that follow will cover what you should be eating, how to make the best food choices, and meal composition, and will provide you with two weeks of meal plans and simply delicious recipes from Dr. Roni's kitchen that make incorporating more live foods into your diet a treat. The balance of the book will describe the nutritional philosophy that will become your culinary way of life.

EATING OUT DOES NOT HAVE TO BE A DISASTER

You can eat healthy when you eat out. You have to make the right choices. It is not as difficult as it used to be. Many restaurants now are health conscious and offer vegetarian and spa cuisine options on their menus. Even fast-food restaurants have healthier choices.

To avoid temptation, skip the bread basket. You can turn it down. Just say no, and the bread will be taken away. If you are with others who want the bread, there is not much you can do. Do your best to restrain yourself. If you are not able to resist, make sure to eat only multigrain or whole-grain bread. You do not have to eat an entire piece—you can try a bite or a piece of the crust.

Ordering a salad is a great way to add some greens and raw vegetables to your meal. If you start with a salad, it will fill you up and you will be less likely to overeat when the main course arrives. Europeans eat their salads after the main course. The size of their portions is much smaller than what is served in America. If you limit your portions, you can fill up on salad after your main course and stay full longer. Either way works. Always ask for dressing on the side. If the dressing is made with olive oil, you can splurge a little. Just make certain no salt or sugar is used. In a pinch, you can dress your salad with balsamic vinegar or other types of vinegar or lemon.

Soup can be a good substitute for a main course, the heartier the better. Just make certain it does not have a cream base. Manhattan clam chowder, yes; New England clam chowder, no. Try to skip soups with rice or noodles, but if you cannot, you do not have to clean your bowl to the bottom. Leave the simple carbs, including potatoes!

Dr. Roni on Drinking with Meals

Try not to drink beverages—even water—while you eat. Digestion begins in your mouth well before food reaches your stomach. The salivary glands, located under your tongue near the lower jaw, produce saliva. Saliva not only moistens the food as you chew, but it also produces amylase, an enzyme that begins to digest the starch and sugar in the food you are eating. Drinking with food dilutes the strength of digestive enzymes in your mouth and stomach. Low enzymes are the third highest digestive problem.

Chew your food well and do not wash your meal down with fluids. Always take an enzyme pill when you eat a meal that requires chewing. Let your body do the work it is supposed to do. I suggest that you drink an hour after meals.

Most chefs are willing to cook without butter and oil, sugar, flour, and salt. Always ask if your food can be prepared with a little olive oil. Chefs will often be willing to prepare something for you that is not on the menu. Simple food is the way to go. Your best bet is to order grilled, poached, or steamed chicken, fish, or shellfish and steamed vegetables. Many restaurants now serve brown rice and whole wheat or whole-grain pasta. Avoid heavy sauces and use lemon for flavor instead. If you are served a large portion, you do not have to eat it all. Do not hesitate to ask your server to pack up what is left. It will make a great lunch the next day.

Have a cup of tea for dessert. Some restaurants will serve plain yogurt on the side. You should avoid ordering fruit for dessert. You will learn why in Chapter 12. For the sake of your digestion, fruit should be eaten alone, two hours before or after a meal.

The meal we have described is delicious and satisfying. You will have little trouble following Dr. Roni's Healthy Eating Plan when you go out to eat. And remember, there is the 75/25 solution to fall back on if you just have to have those BBQ ribs.

STAYING ON TRACK AT PARTIES

The best advice we can give you about eating well at parties is to have a protein shake before you go. Never go to a party hungry. Hors d'oeuvres and finger food can be a great temptation. They seem so little and harmless, but they can be packed with butter, oils, salt, cream, and ingredients you want to avoid. Go for live foods—crudités are always a good option. Skip the chips, pretzels, and creamy dips. A handful of unsalted nuts will carry you. Whole-grain crackers or crudités with some hummus will see you through. Shrimp cocktail is fine. Take an enzyme tablet with your club soda with a squeeze of fresh lemon or lime to help digest your food. It is best not to drink wine or mixed drinks at a party, because you will tend to eat more when your inhibitions relax.

Try eating a "mono meal." Just eat one type of food—the meat, poultry, or fish; the vegetables—or the potatoes, bread, and sweets if you want to indulge. The last thing you want to do is overtax your digestive system by eating a wild variety of foods. If you eat only one food type, you are not likely to overeat.

Once again, you might choose an occasional party as part of your 25 percent time off from Dr. Roni's Healthy Eating Plan. If you are at a friend's wedding, you may not want to skip the champagne toast and wedding cake. When officemates go to the trouble of getting you a birthday cake, it would be rude not to take a slice—though you do not have to eat all of it. Those brisket sandwiches at a tailgate party might be irresistible. Parties are for celebrating, and if you feel like celebrating, go for it. But remember, these indulgences have to remain an aberration, not the norm.

HOW TO SURVIVE THE HOLIDAYS WITHOUT GAINING TEN POUNDS

One of the best ways to avoid gaining weight during the holidays is to schedule a detox one week or weekend prior to the holiday. Follow the plans in Chapter 14. Many regular detoxers do the full detox after New Year's Day to correct the overeating of the holiday season and to start the year off right.

During holidays, we recommend practicing many of the at home therapies described in Chapter 8. Getting some time in an infrared sauna, doing the dry skin brush, or having a coffee enema will help. You should drink a lot of distilled water, which will clean you out. If you add lemon or vinegar to the water, you will reduce acidity and make your body more alkaline. Take brisk walks every day. You might want to try taking magnesium at night. Make sure to take an enzyme pill whenever you eat. Do whatever you can to help your body expel toxins you might be consuming.

If you are facing big feasts, try the mono meal strategy. Eat all the meat served, exclusively, or all the side vegetables. If you want a carb binge, now is the time, but eat *only* carbohydrates. By not mixing food groups, you will not overstress your digestive system. If you cannot resist that grilled cheeseburger on a toasted bun and corn on the cob slathered in butter at the July Fourth picnic, enjoy it. Just be ready to eat clean when the holiday is over.

FOOD CRAVINGS DO NOT HAVE TO RULE YOU

Everyone craves food now and then. The urge to eat potato chips, chocolate, french fries, ice cream, or chocolate chip cookies is common. Sometimes food cravings can signal a nutritional need. When you are on the nutrient-dense diet of Dr. Roni's Healthy Eating Plan this should not be a problem, because your body's needs are being met. More often, food cravings are the desire for a particular feeling or result—like a sugar rush from eating candy. Then there are comfort foods that satisfy emotional needs, calming stress and reducing anxiety.

Some cravings are habits or food addictions. Scientists have found that food cravings activate the same reward pathways in the brain as cravings for drugs and alcohol. If you continually eat high-sugar, high-fat foods, many of the dopamine receptors in your reward pathways shut down to prevent overload. Dopamine is a neurotransmitter that is responsible for reward-driven learning. When fewer dopamine receptors are at work, the system craves more and more, and one cookie is not enough. When that happens, you develop food addictions. Food addictions cause changes in parts of the brain that normally override impulses and addictive cravings.

There is a good chance that you have conquered your food addictions during the detox, but emotional triggers can set off the craving pattern again. When you feel a food craving intensely, it is sometimes good to give in to it. Deprivation can make the craving stronger. We are not talking about bingeing, but a few fast-food french fries might satisfy you. Do not eat the entire portion. A piece of 70% cacao chocolate is actually good for you. An occasional slice of pizza is fine, but do not devour an entire pie loaded with pepperoni and meatballs.

Drinking water or seltzer with flavored stevia can satisfy a sweet tooth. Exercise can cut food cravings. If you have an excessive craving for sweets, you can try sugar-controlling herbs. We recommend taking Glucofast, which is good if you are insulin resistant. You can check out the website www.hellolife.glucofast.net.

Another helpful technique involves postponing gratification. When you crave a particular food, set a timer for thirty minutes and divert yourself with something else. Do a chore, make a phone call, surf the Internet. When the thirty minutes are up, the craving might have passed. If you can delay eating the food you crave, you can weaken the habitual response. The longer you curb your cravings, the weaker the urges become.

If you are eating in response to feelings, you have to examine those emotions. Consider honestly whether indulging in junk food is really making you feel better. Eating unhealthy food is certainly not solving the problem. When you have a food craving, write in your journal about what you crave and what is going on in your life that might be fueling the urge for comfort. Examine the feelings stressful situations evoke. Analyzing a craving this way can make

How to Handle Food Cravings

Drink water with fresh lemon, lime, or flavored stevia.

Exercise or take a walk for thirty minutes.

Write in your journal about what you are feeling and why you crave comfort food.

Meditate or do yoga to relieve the stress that is behind the craving.

Set a timer for thirty minutes and distract yourself by making a phone call, surfing the Internet, or doing a chore.

Take a sugar-controlling herbs like Glucofast.

When all else fails, give in and have a small portion of what you crave.

it go away. Try yoga or meditation to deal with the stress behind the impulse to find comfort in food. If you cannot control your emotional eating or food addictions, you might want to seek professional help or join Food Addicts Anonymous (www.foodaddicts anonymous.org) to see a food addiction counselor.

STAY LIGHT FOREVER

We want to give you the tools and the knowledge to make healthy food choices from the huge range of possibilities out there. We also want you to understand how your body works and what you can do to keep it in prime working order. Dr. Roni's Healthy Eating Plan will take the guesswork out of how to eat to stay slim, energized, and glowing. The next chapter will show you how to eat clean for the rest of your life.

Detox Success Story
I LEARNED TO LISTEN TO MY BODY

I'm twenty-eight years old and have struggled with my weight for ten years. I was diagnosed with juvenile rheumatoid arthritis at age sixteen and have had a ten-year-long battle with sinus and allergy issues. While in college, I gained thirty pounds. I got the weight off using diet and exercise within a year and a half of graduation. At age twenty-one, I was diagnosed with fibromyalgia, and at twenty-four with Behcet's syndrome, an autoimmune disorder. When I got diagnosed with Behcet's, I was on a downward spiral physically, mentally, and emotionally.

I had been taking steroids for a long time, so all the weight came back. I lost twenty to twenty-five pounds again with diet and exercise. Shortly after losing the weight, I tore a muscle while preparing for a half marathon and was unable to exercise for several months. I kept my weight stable without running. Then after some family issues, I started to put the weight back on again. I was five pounds away from my highest weight ever, and I knew that I needed to make drastic changes in my lifestyle. I decided to detox and to educate myself on the principles of food combining and the link between physical, mental, and emotional health.

I read Dr. Roni's first book in 2008 and decided there was no way I could stick to such a rigid plan. I put the book back on the shelf, and there it sat for four years. I read it again in January 2012 and decided to take the plunge, because I was ready to lose weight and get my energy and self-confidence back.

When I started the detox, I was five feet, seven inches and 163 pounds. I felt overweight and mentally and physically worn down, because I had let my health and wellness decline for so long. I started the detox the day after Easter. It was perfect timing, heading into spring. I definitely had my ups and downs throughout the detox, but I started feeling great by Day 4. I was already noting brighter skin and a flatter stomach. By Day 6, others were telling me that I looked thinner. I noticed a major decrease in my cellulite. By Day 7, I was already down ten pounds. By Day 10, all my clothes were loose. I no longer experienced my midafternoon slumps.

My attitude changed immensely! I believe that this was due to the fact that my physical health was improving. I felt empowered by my ability to follow a plan and stick to it. It was exhilarating to know that I could go to business lunch meetings, cocktail hours, sporting events, and birthday celebrations and still stick to the plan in order to improve my health. About halfway through the detox, I noticed that I wasn't feeling deprived or like I was missing out when I wasn't enjoying the food and wine at various events.

I lost fifteen pounds in fifteen days, and an additional three pounds. I noticed three major changes in my health. My allergies disappeared and I started to sleep through the night. Lastly, I learned to listen to my body. I felt so great during the detox that I wanted to keep that feeling going. When I'm not detoxing, I know right away when I'm not treating my body right or when it is time to get a colonic. I still use the berry drink, green drink, aloe vera, probiotics, sauna treatments, skin brushing, and colonics as part of my normal health and wellness routine.

Amy Guerich

CHAPTER 11

~

EAT CLEAN

Many Americans organize their lives around food. We have power breakfasts, hold meetings over lunch, hit the free buffet at happy hour, celebrate birthdays and holidays with special meals. Our toxic food environment makes changing eating habits a challenge. Wherever we turn, junk food is everywhere—at the gas station, in vending machines, at the newsstand in the lobby. It is easy to become an emotional eater, hooked on sweets and processed carbs, or a food addict.

So many factors contribute to weight gain. Losing weight and keeping it off cannot be reduced to calories in/calories out. Here are just a few factors at play:

- The extent to which toxins interfere with your bodily processes and have compromised your body
- How efficiently your body digests certain foods, including processed foods, grains, sweets, and fruits
- The types of grains and starchy carbohydrates that you eat
- Whether your body diverts extra calories into your muscles for energy or into your fat cells for storage
- How well your body processes insulin, which transports glucose out of the bloodstream and into the cells for energy
- Whether the foods you eat contain enough enzymes

Any of these issues can compromise your metabolism and prevent you from losing weight. Dr. Roni's Healthy Eating Plan takes care of these issues.

You are one of the lucky few. Having completed your detox and transition, you are beginning with a clean slate. You have made your gradual transition from the detox. You need to carry over what you have learned and avoid returning to your prior eating habits. This chapter is a crash course in good nutrition. Our intention is to give you a sense of the rich array of foods you will be eating that will maintain your weight loss and keep your body functioning at peak performance.

KEEP A HEALTHY EATING LOG

Now that you are establishing new eating habits, recording what you eat each day is a good way to stay mindful of how good your food choices are. Make sure to note when you take your supplements, how many glasses of water you drink, and how much exercise you get each day.

You can also make note of when you get hungry, if you do. You will then be able to see patterns and adjust what you are eating. You should note any food cravings that pop up as well.

Keeping a record of your energy level at different points of the day can reveal whether your body is getting adequate nutrition. Here is an idea of what you should include on a log page.

The Problem with Salt

Packaged food manufacturers mask the lack of flavor in refined foods by adding lots of salt or sodium. If you eat processed foods, it is important to read the nutritional label. Many contain between 25 and 45 percent of the maximum salt intake recommended each day: 2,400 milligrams, which is about one teaspoon of salt a day.

If you are like most people, once you cut back on your salt, you will notice your body change. Any bloating will go down, foot and ankle swelling will subside, and your blood pressure will drop. Cut back on salt before talking to your doctor about reducing or eliminating your blood pressure medication.

HEALTHY EATING LOG

Hours of Sleep Last Night:

State of Mind at Start of the Day:

TIME	MEAL	LEVEL OF HUNGER
Breakfast		
Snack		
Lunch		
Snack		
Dinner		
Nighttime Snack		
8 oz. water	O O O O O O O O	
Exercise		
Relaxation/Restoration (what time did I take for myself?)		
Peak Energy of Day (time)		
Lowest Energy of Day (time)		

You do not need to keep a log forever. That would be unrealistic. Why not keep a log for forty days? They say that forty days is enough time to break a habit. At the beginning of your return to post-detox eating, it will help you as you begin to eat your new everyday diet. Just make forty copies of this log page to record what you eat each day and how you feel. Being mindful of how you are eating will help you change.

EAT NATURAL, WHOLE FOODS

Whole foods are not adulterated in any way. Superior to highly processed foods, they contain all their original nutrients. They do not need to be refined or enriched. Whole foods have the enzymes necessary for your body to digest and absorb nutrients. The processed foods you find packaged in the center aisles of the supermarket lose many nutrients in processing. Chemicals are added to the food to replace natural nutrients that have been lost in the process. You already know that your body has a hard time digesting and using food filled with preservatives, additives, and dyes.

If you eat processed foods, you are not nourishing your body well. When your body is starved for nutrients, you will keep eating until it obtains what it needs. The more low-quality food you eat, the more you will want to eat. That can undo all the work you have done. You do not want to reintroduce processed foods into your diet now. The idea is not to open a can, bag, or box for food. Frozen unprocessed food is fine. In fact, having frozen berries for smoothies is a good idea.

Whole Grains

There is no place for refined white flour in your diet. All the nutrition has been stripped from the grain as the bran is milled from the outside of the wheat. The same is true for white rice. You have to shift to eating only whole grains. Whole grains are the seeds of a plant and contain the nutrients and energy to support the growth of the plant.

There are many benefits to eating whole grains. The fiber helps to lower cholesterol and puts the absorption of glucose on a time delay, so you do not get a sugar high or spike in your blood sugar. The vitamin E in whole grains prevents LDL cholesterol from reacting with oxygen to clog your arteries. The layer of bran in whole grains supplies magnesium, selenium, copper, and manganese. Studies have shown that whole grains reduce the risk of heart disease, stroke, cancer, diabetes, and obesity.

Incorporating whole grains into your diet should be easy. Substitute brown rice for white rice, and whole wheat or whole-grain pasta for white flour pasta. Whole grains are a source of protein. Quinoa, for example, contains all of the essential amino acids, which are the building blocks of protein. Experiment with quinoa, amaranth, barley, buckwheat, bulgur, and whole wheat couscous. You can use them in soups or as a pasta substitute. Have steel-cut oats for breakfast rather than instant oatmeal. Steel-cut oats will keep you feeling fuller, because they are digested more slowly.

Load Up on the Vegetables and Fruit

One-half to three-quarters of what you eat should be living foods, packed with enzymes and phytonutrients. That means shopping at the perimeter of the grocery store for fresh produce. At this point, you do not need to be convinced of the importance of incorporating many servings of vegetables into your diet. You will continue to drink freshly squeezed juices and powdered green juices on Dr. Roni's Healthy Eating Plan. Now that you can chew again, you can enjoy a full range of vegetables and salads. The chart that follows will show you the nutritional gifts of eating the rainbow.

Eat by Color

One extremely healthy way to eat is to select vegetables with colors that span the spectrum from the deepest violet to the brightest white. Each color corresponds to a different set of phytonutrients, natural compounds that are found in foods that work alongside vitamins and minerals to promote good health.

COLOR	VEGETABLE	PHYTONUTRIENT
White	Garlic, onions, cauliflower, jicama, parsnips, turnips, onions	Alum, allicin
Yellow/orange	Carrots, summer squash, sweet potatoes, yams	Beta-carotene, bioflavonoids, vitamins A and C, potassium
Red	Red cabbage, red onions, red peppers, tomatoes, beets, radishes	Vitamin C, lycopene, anthocyanins
Purple	Purple endive (radicchio), eggplant, red cabbage	Phenolics, anthocyanins
Green	Broccoli, celery, cucumbers, kale, collards, chard, spinach, other greens	Indoles, lutein, potassium, vitamin K, zeaxanthin
Brown	Sea vegetables like dried algae, kelp, and kombu	Iodine, vitamin K, folate, magnesium, iron

Organic Produce

In the second part of this book, we discussed the importance of eating organic produce. Organic food is grown without poisons or hormones. More than 400 chemical pesticides are routinely used in conventional farming. Residues of those poisons remain on commercially raised produce even after washing. You will remember that these pesticides are endocrine disrupters, which remain in your body long after you eat. Be certain to wash all fruits and vegetables—even organic produce—thoroughly.

Organic food is usually 20 percent more expensive than chemically grown food. In weighing the price difference, you have to consider the cost of the potential health damage to yourself and your family. With your newly sensitized taste buds, you will appreciate the superior flavor of organic food. Buying organic produce is good for the planet, as we explained earlier.

If you have trouble finding organic produce or do not want to buy only organic produce, you can make choices about lowering your pesticide intake. The Environmental Work Group compiles lists each year rating the pesticide levels of fruits and vegetables. The first list has those with the highest levels of pesticides and other toxins. Buy the produce on this list organic or do not eat it.

THE DIRTY DOZEN

Do your best to avoid conventionally grown fruits and vegetables from this list. It is advisable to buy these foods organic, because they are high in pesticide residues.

1. Apples
2. Celery
3. Strawberries
4. Peaches
5. Spinach
6. Nectarines
7. Grapes
8. Sweet bell peppers
9. Potatoes
10. Blueberries
11. Lettuce
12. Kale/collard greens

THE CLEAN FIFTEEN

These are the fruits and vegetables with the lowest levels of pesticides. If you have to make a choice, this is the produce you can buy conventionally grown.

1. Onions
2. Sweet corn (not grown from genetically modified seeds)
3. Pineapples
4. Avocado
5. Asparagus

6. Sweet peas
7. Mangoes
8. Eggplant
9. Cantaloupe
10. Kiwi
11. Cabbage
12. Watermelon
13. Sweet potatoes
14. Grapefruit
15. Mushrooms

Animals, Fish, and Shellfish

You have already learned that a diet high in animal fat is not good for you, particularly if the beef, poultry, and pork were raised on feedlots with antibiotics and growth hormones. Buy free-range, organically raised meat. We recommend that you eat animal protein sparingly, no more than three times a week, and when you do, consume meat with the lowest fat content available. That means eating poultry without the skin, unless the meal falls in your 25 percent zone.

Dr. Roni's Meat Warning

Eating animal protein is not bad in and of itself. What is unhealthy about red meat is the amount of saturated fat some varieties contain. When you shop for any type of meat, poultry, or fish, be sure to choose the leanest cuts and slice off the fat or skin before you eat. Choose cuts from grass-fed animals, which are leaner and cleaner than conventional products and do not contain antibiotics and hormones.

Avoid prime cuts when you buy beef. They are loaded with fat. Buy the lowest fat content you can find for ground beef, turkey, and chicken. For pork and lamb, tenderloin, loin chops, and leg are good choices. When buying turkey or chicken, select breasts over thighs and always remove the skin.

If you cannot resist a thick, juicy steak, enjoy it. Drink green juice the next day.

Fish and shellfish have always been considered a great source of protein. Fish contains omega-3 fatty acids, vitamin D, and iodine. But today, much of our seafood is contaminated by mercury and other heavy metals. Mercury accumulates up the food chain in fish and shellfish, so large predatory fish at the top of the chain live longer and contain higher levels of mercury. Mercury is stored in fat tissue, the brain, and the bones. Ridding your body of mercury takes several months. Its half-life is about eighty days.

You want to eat fish with the lowest mercury content. The Natural Resources Defense Council (NRDC) has rated the mercury levels in a comprehensive list of fish, which is reproduced below as a reference. Fish is a staple of our diets on the Vineyard, so we are giving you the complete list. You should try to eat fish that have the lowest levels of mercury.

Mercury Levels in Fish

HIGHEST MERCURY LEVELS

King mackerel	Shark
Marlin	Swordfish
Orange roughy	Tuna (ahi, bigeye)

HIGH MERCURY LEVELS

Bluefish	Mackerel (Spanish, gulf)
Chilean sea bass	Tuna (canned white
Grouper	albacore, yellowfin)

LOWER MERCURY LEVELS

Bass (striped, black)	Perch (freshwater)
Carp	Sablefish
Cod	Sea trout
Croaker	Skate
Halibut	Snapper
Lobster	Tuna (canned chunk
Mahimahi	light)
Monkfish	

LOWEST MERCURY LEVELS

Anchovies	Crayfish
Butterfish	Croaker
Catfish	Flounder
Clams	Haddock
Crab	Hake

Herring	Scallops
Mackerel (North Atlantic, chub)	Shad
	Shrimp
Mullet	Sole
Oysters	Squid
Perch (ocean)	Tilapia
Plaice	Trout (freshwater)
Salmon (canned, fresh)	Whitefish
Sardines	Whiting

The choice of fish with the lowest mercury levels is extensive. Fish is part of your restricted animal protein. On Dr. Roni's Healthy Eating Plan, you have three portions of fish, meat, or poultry, a week.

Good Fats

Essential fatty acids (EFAs) omega-3 and omega-6 are polyunsaturated fats that cannot be produced by the body. These fats must be obtained from your diet.

They have a critical role in health and disease prevention. EFAs support the cardiovascular, immune, nervous and reproductive systems. Though consumption of omega-3 should be equal to four times greater than consumption of omega-6, most Americans consume ten to twenty-five times more omega-6 than omega-3. Omega-3s are used in the formation of cell walls, making them supple and flexible and enabling the cells to absorb maximum nutrition and expel harmful waste products. Omega-3 deficiency is very common. Omega-3 deficiencies are linked to decreased memory and mental abilities, tingling sensations of the nerves, poor vision, blood clots, diminished immune function, increased triglycerides and bad cholesterol, hypertension, and menopausal discomfort. Omega-3 is found in:

Flaxseed oil, flaxseeds, flaxseed meal
Hempseed oil and hemp seeds

Walnuts
    Pumpkin seeds
    Brazil nuts
    Sesame seeds
    Avocados
    Dark leafy green vegetables (kale, spinach, purslane,
        mustard greens, collards, chard)
    Cold pressed, unrefined canola oil
    Salmon
    Mackerel
    Sardines
    Anchovies

To keep your cells healthy and prevent illness, make sure you are eating foods rich in omega-3 fatty acids.

PICK YOUR POISON: ARTIFICIAL SWEETENERS

Many people use sugar substitutes to reduce calories and help maintain or lose weight. Artificial sweeteners are "plastic foods"—man-made food-like substances that manufacturers try to convince us are good for us but in reality are good only for them. Here is Dr. Roni's rule of thumb about food labels: If you do not know what the ingredient is, neither will your body, so consider it toxic. The chemicals aspartame, acesulfame, neotame, sucralose, and alitame—more commonly known as NutraSweet and Equal in the blue packages, Splenda in yellow packages, Sweet 'N Low and saccharin in pink packages—all fall on that list. Your body just does not know how to process these synthetic substances.

The zero-calorie sweetener of preference is stevia, made from a South American herb. You can buy it in liquid or powdered form in health food stores and most supermarkets. It is available in green packages in health food restaurants. Stevia is more than thirty times sweeter than sugar, so you do not need to use much. It does not cause your blood sugar to spike or cause the cravings that other sugars do. It does have an aftertaste that you will have to get accustomed to.

If you cannot find stevia, try a natural, complex sweetener like agave nectar, raw honey, maple syrup, or molasses. These cause glucose to enter the bloodstream, but at a slower pace than when you consume sugar or high fructose corn syrup.

And stay away from high fructose corn syrup at all costs. This means eliminating most processed foods.

EAT TO FIGHT INFLAMMATION

Inflammation is increasingly seen to underlie many age-related diseases and to be at the root of aging itself. Junk food, fast food, sugar, high-fat meats, saturated fats and trans fats used in prepared and processed foods, and nitrates found in hot dogs, cold cuts, and sausages promote inflammation. To quiet chronic inflammation, inhibit oxidative stress, and boost your immune system, your body needs essential amino acids, linoleic acid (an essential fatty acid), vitamin A, folic acid, vitamins B_6 and B_{12}, vitamin C, vitamin E, zinc, copper, iron, and selenium. Deficiencies in one or more of these nutrients can increase inflammation. When your body becomes inflamed on a cellular level, the aging process accelerates. It is important to be aware of the foods that fight inflammation when you choose what you eat.

> Aside from the fact that my skin was glowing and my hair was shining when I finished the detox, I was standing up straighter and moving more fluidly, since my joints were not inflamed. That was a gigantic change.
>
> Melissa Scarry

Anti-Inflammatory Foods

Making sure you eat food that fights inflammation will slow down the aging process and prevent diseases associated with aging. These are the foods you should chose from.

> **Vegetables:** Arugula, asparagus, bean sprouts, bell pepper, bok choy, broccoli, broccoli rabe, Brussels sprouts, cabbage, cauliflower, chard, collards, cucumber, endive, escarole, garlic, green beans, kale, leek, mushrooms, olives, onion, romaine lettuce, scallions (green onions), shallots, spinach, sweet potato, zucchini
>
> **Fruit:** Apples, avocado, blueberries, cantaloupe, cherries, clementines, guava, honeydew, kiwifruit, kumquats, lemon, lime, orange, papaya, peaches, pears, plums, raspberries, rhubarb, strawberries, tangerines, tomato
>
> **Animal protein (grass-fed or wild preferred):** Anchovies, skinless and boneless chicken breast, oysters, rainbow trout, salmon, sardines, shad, turkey breast
>
> **Nuts and seeds:** Almonds, flaxseeds, hazelnuts, sunflower seeds, walnuts
>
> **Oils:** Extra-virgin olive oil, flaxseed oil
>
> **Herbs and spices:** ginger, oregano, turmeric
>
> **Drinks:** Green tea, ginger tea

WHAT TO DO WHEN YOU HAVE THE NIBBLES

Snacks are what undermine most diets. Now that you have dropped processed foods, you may be at a loss about what to munch on when you need a snack. Here are some ideas for some snacks that are as healthy as they are tasty:

> Chopped raw green beans and almonds
> ¼ cup unsalted raw nuts
> Avocado on cucumber slices

Almond butter on cucumber slices

1 cup of organic mixed berries

Hummus on celery sticks

6 ounces Greek-style yogurt with vanilla extract and
cinnamon sprinkles

Raw veggie sticks with almond or cashew butter

Apple or pear slices dipped in cinnamon

Blueberries with chopped basil and balsamic vinegar

Two pieces deviled egg (1 egg)

Hot cocoa protein shake

2 ounces of tuna salad wrapped in a large piece of lettuce
(buy organic mayonnaise or make your own; recipe on
page 246.)

Egg salad wrapped in large spinach leaves (use organic or
homemade mayonnaise)

Salmon salad on raw onion or cucumber slices (use organic
or homemade mayonnaise)

Baked sweet potato topped with chopped walnuts

½ cup cottage cheese with flaxseed oil and diced tomatoes

Edamame

You get the idea. You have to think outside the box. You are no longer reaching for a bag of chips or a couple of cookies. Snacks are a good time to increase your vegetable and fruit intake. If you cannot live without crackers, look for ones that are gluten free and made from whole grains, and eat them sparingly.

*   *   *

To summarize the principles of good eating covered in this chapter, here are Dr. Roni's basic rules of nutrition for optimal health.

- Take maximum nutrition in small doses.
- Eat only natural foods.
- Eat only whole foods.

- Eat primarily living foods—50 to 75 percent of your diet.
- Eat only poison-free foods.
- Eat only sugar-free foods (without sucrose and fructose).
- Do not use table salt. Natural sodium is found in vegetables, fruit, fish, and seafood.

Your high energy and high spirits will make following these guidelines a breeze. Eating this way will become a habit you will not want to break.

Detox Success Story

I STOPPED LOOKING IN THE MIRROR, AND I SHOPPED FOR SHOES

It started with a kiss, a birthday wish, and a gift of the book *21 Pounds in 21 Days*. So what kind of a gift is this? I see it worked for you, the gift giver, but you know me, I've done them all, and I'm not your age—I'm much older and much more tired of trying things that don't work for me. This was October 2009. Size 16W. Age 59.

I had given up, given away my prized items that would never fit again. I stopped looking in the mirror, and I shopped for shoes. And the book sat on my table for eight months, I glanced at it, dusted the cover as needed, put it out of my mind.

Late June 2010, I was on a vacation, feeling upset I wasn't putting on a bathing suit, really looking at myself, feeling just old. I decided right there and then to go for it. And I did.

I had a tired feeling and chills by the third day, referred to in the book as a healing crisis, and that passed quickly. I started to feel so much better by Day 4 and the feeling just grew. I didn't want to sleep, I wanted to stay up late, rise early, and keep moving.

I have a lot to lose, and at my age I didn't expect to lose twenty-one pounds at all. A process started, it was summer, I was slimming down. It was noticeable. My skin glowed, and everyone told me so. I stopped eating meat as a result of this initial cleansing process.

I started the second detox soon after, with summer in full swing, taking advantage of the hot days and abundance of sunlight to keep me going, and it did. Everyone took notice. I actually had to buy a few different items to wear.

Oh, yes, I went for a third by Halloween. I was on a roll.

By December 2010, I was off Crestor; my labs were perfect, and my MD complimented me, asking for details about the detox, colonics, and coffee enemas, all that I had continued during my maintenance phase.

Reading the book, looking in the mirror, drinking my nutrients on time, reading comments from others on the journey, keeping busy, and being positive helped me stay the course.

Overall, I am more mindful about what I eat. Portions are the issue and have been so. What I ingest is very different. Still, I'm not eating meat. I'm having whole wheat pasta instead, lots of veggies and nuts and beans and quinoa as well as my Bragg Liquid Aminos in everything. And yes, I still have my drinks when I'm on maintenance and thereafter. That's always.

I am addicted to sugar. When I relapse, I get a serious brain fog, reminding me to stop and get back on track, so I do. I also don't allow more than a five-pound weight gain, because now I actually know what five pounds feel and look like.

When I detox, I go for the gusto, the full twenty-one days. And for me, each one is different. Sometimes it's so easy, and other times, I feel challenged. When it's easy, I go for another one, because for some reason my metabolism is working so much better.

At least twelve people I know have considered detoxing with me. They have not followed through as of yet, even though they bought the book and check the Facebook page. I'm not sure why, but I do recall all those months I walked by the book without turning a page.

October 2012. Size 8P. Age 62.

As of this writing, I'm detoxing again, enjoying my chills, my energy (I work at a full-time and a part-time job), going out dancing at least two times a month, up until midnight, rising at 6:00 a.m., loving my sauna and my steam and just wishing I had more time to get to the gym!!!

Life, Be It, and now, I truly am.

Patti Firrincili

CHAPTER 12

〜

THE BALANCING ACT

Though the demands of your never-a-dull-moment life can stress you out, there is a way to stay centered. Physical, mental, and emotional imbalance is rooted in the chemical balance of your cells. If the chemical balance of your body is off, the result goes beyond physical disease. Your emotions and spirit will be thrown out of whack, too.

The body has a built-in drive to achieve homeostasis, or balance. The fluids in your body are acid, neutral, or alkaline. Your pH balance indicates how acidic or alkaline your body is. On a scale of 0 to 14, the ideal neutral pH balance is between 6.5 and 7.0. A pH level less than 7 is considered acidic; greater than 7 is base or alkaline. Your cells function at their peak when your pH is slightly alkaline.

Activity between your cells is controlled by pH, which regulates your digestive system and determines how your body uses enzymes, minerals, and vitamins. The normal pH for all tissues and fluids is alkaline, except for the stomach, which produces acidic enzymes for digestion. When your body converts food to energy, the process creates by-products that can be acidic. The standard American diet promotes excess acidity. Coffee, processed foods, dairy products, and a lack of fresh produce all contribute to an acidic state. If acid levels in your body become too high, your organs of elimination have a hard time flushing out the acid. An acidic internal environment leads to degeneration and disease. The signs and symptoms of pH imbalance can be subtle and nonspecific. You may feel fatigued and lethargic. The symptoms associated with having an acid body include:

Weight gain
Obesity
Loss of elasticity in the skin,
    also known as wrinkles
Loss of vitality
Chronic fatigue
Joint pain
Aching muscles
Stomachache
Ulcers
Nausea
Urinary-tract problems
Kidney stones
Constipation
Gout
Osteopenia and osteoporosis
Immune deficiency
Constriction of blood vessels
Circulatory and
    cardiovascular weakness

> I have learned to use pH balance foods to reduce dietary inflammation and thereby reduce overall stress on my body. As a result, I don't eat much meat anymore (fish once a week) and get my protein from plant sources. Not on any antianxiety meds anymore and fifteen pounds lighter. I have not been sustainable at this weight, ever. I am a triathlete, so every pound helps reduce joint damage over the years. Thanks for being the catalyst that started my new health regimen.
>
> L.R.

There is a limit to what your body can do to reverse overacidity, but you can balance your pH through your diet. What you eat supports or detracts from your equilibrium, which has a direct effect on every aspect of your physical, mental, emotional, and spiritual health.

Most refined foods lower the body's pH, making it more acidic. Acidic biochemistry contributes to weak teeth and bone loss, because the body scavenges vital minerals from our bones and teeth in an attempt to bring the body into balance. There is a link between common overly acidic foods and societal epidemics like obesity, hypertension, high cholesterol, and diabetes. The key to alkalizing nutrition is to eat fruits and vegetables that are rich in enzymes. These are the steps you need to take to reduce the acidity in your body:

- Avoid white sugar.
- Decrease the amount of fat you consume.
- Eat less meat.
- Eat more nuts, seeds, and whole grains.
- Eat more fruits and vegetables, especially raw for maximum nutrition.
- Use fresh lemon.

Sound familiar? Dr. Roni's Healthy Eating Plan will help you to alkalize your body.

For quick reference, we are including a chart that will give you a picture of which foods are acidic and alkaline and to what degree.

ACID- AND ALKALINE-FORMING FOODS

MOST ACIDIC	ACIDIC	LOW ACID	LOW ALKALINE	ALKALINE	MOST ALKALINE
SWEETENERS					
NutraSweet, Equal, Aspartame, Sweet 'N Low	White sugar, brown sugar	Processed honey, molasses	Raw honey, raw sugar	Maple syrup	Stevia
FRUITS					
Blueberries, cranberries, prunes	Sour cherries, rhubarb, unripe fruit	Plums, processed fruit juices	Oranges, bananas, cherries, pineapple, peaches, avocados	Dates, figs, melons, kiwifruit, berries, apples, pears, raisins	Lemons, watermelon, limes, grapefruit, mangoes, papayas

VEGETABLES					
Sauerkraut	Skinless potatoes, pinto beans, navy beans, lima beans	Cooked spinach, green beans, kidney beans	Carrots, tomatoes, fresh corn, mushrooms, cabbage, peas, potato skins, olives, soybeans, tofu	Okra, squash, green beans, beets, celery, lettuce, zucchini, sweet potato	Asparagus, onion, fresh vegetable juices, parsley, leaf spinach, broccoli, swiss chard
NUTS AND SEEDS					
Peanuts, walnuts	Pecans, cashews	Pumpkin seeds, sunflower seeds	Chestnuts	Almonds	
FATS AND OILS					
Processed oils		Corn oil	Canola oil	Flaxseed oil	Olive oil
GRAINS AND GRAIN PRODUCTS					
Wheat, white flour, pastries, pasta	White rice, corn, buckwheat, oats, rye	Sprouted wheat bread, spelt, brown rice	Amaranth, millet, wild rice		
MEAT, POULTRY, AND FISH					
Beef, pork, shellfish	Turkey, chicken, lamb	Venison, cold-water fish			
DAIRY PRODUCTS					
Cheese, pasteurized milk, ice cream, chocolate	Eggs, butter, yogurt, buttermilk, cottage cheese	Raw milk, whey, soy cheese, soy milk, goat milk, goat cheese			
BEVERAGES					
Beer, soft drinks	Coffee, alcohol	Tea	Ginger tea	Green tea	Herb teas, lemon and hot water

When you are constructing a meal, the ideal balance is 80 percent alkaline-forming foods and 20 percent acid-forming foods. The best quick fixes to move your pH balance to alkaline are to squeeze fresh lemon into the water you drink during the day and to drink a green juice, either fresh or powdered. Dr. Roni has you covered.

ANOTHER BALANCING ACT: KEEPING YOUR BLOOD SUGAR LEVEL

The demand for energy in your body never stops. Your brain in particular requires an even supply of glucose to function at its best. The glucose level in your bloodstream is regulated by a hormone balancing act involving insulin and glucagon. Insulin is responsible for taking excess energy and storing it as fat, and glucagon mobilizes energy. Insulin drives down blood sugar levels by stimulating cells to absorb the glucose carried in the bloodstream and to store it as fat. If the glucose levels in your blood go below a critical level, your brain will signal for more glucose. If glucose is not delivered to your hungry brain, your mind tunes out and you experience mental fatigue and a dramatic mood change called hypoglycemia (low blood sugar). Hypoglycemia can lead to fatigue, irritability, palpitations, headaches, anxiety, difficulty concentrating, paleness, and shakiness. One way to avoid this condition is to eat several small meals to keep your blood sugar stable. This is one of the reasons Dr. Roni's Healthy Eating Plan has you nourishing your body at regular intervals during the day.

When insulin resistance occurs, blood sugar stays at high levels, forcing your pancreas to produce more insulin in an effort to control your high blood sugar levels. If this state continues, insulin-producing cells can wear out, and type 2 diabetes can develop.

You can manage your blood sugar with your diet. The balance between insulin and glucagon is based on the size of a meal and its ratio of carbohydrates to protein. Eating right helps to maintain the hormonal balance to keep your blood sugar at optimal levels.

When you eat simple carbohydrates, your blood sugar rises. How high your blood sugar spikes depends on what you eat, how much you eat, and how much insulin your body produces in response. Glucose then drops quickly and you have the urge to snack. Avoiding refined carbohydrates—white rice or foods made from white flour—will help to keep your blood sugar levels optimal. Processed carbohydrates cause rapid and big increases in blood sugar. Eating whole grains, most fruits and vegetables, and beans produces gradual, smaller, and slower increases.

Easily digested foods cause blood sugar and insulin to spike. The speed with which food is digested is affected by a number of factors. Processing foods often strips the outer protective layer that is hard to digest. The amount of fiber in food slows its digestion. For example, a whole orange with its natural fiber content takes longer to digest than a glass of orange juice. Indigestible fiber carries partially digested food with it while passing through the intestines, so that food is not immediately digested.

Food interactions also affect blood sugar levels. We will discuss food combinations in the next chapter. Fat keeps food in the stomach longer, delaying its entry into the intestines. A food or meal that contains the right fats will keep blood sugar levels down.

The rate at which a carbohydrate enters the bloodstream is called the glycemic index. The lower the glycemic index is, the more slowly the sugar enters the bloodstream and the more consistently the glucose is delivered to your brain. Since food with a low glycemic index breaks down slowly, it has a less dramatic impact on blood sugar and insulin and keeps you feeling full. The glycemic index is determined by the structure of the simple sugars, the fiber content, and the fat content. Understanding the glycemic index of your foods will help you to manage your body's insulin production and minimize insulin resistance. That means your body will burn energy instead of storing it as fat.

Glycemic Index

Glycemic index is measured on a scale of 1 to 100, in which 100 equals pure glucose. The breakdown is as follows:

High glycemic index	70 and above
Medium glycemic index	56–69
Low glycemic index	55 or under

To familiarize you with how this scale applies to the food you eat, we are including a chart of the glycemic index of common foods.

FOOD	RATING	GLYCEMIC INDEX
BREADS AND PASTRIES		
Bagel	High	72
Croissant	Medium	67
Doughnut	High	76
Waffles	High	76
Multigrain bread	Low	48
Whole-grain bread	Low	50
White bread	High	71
White hard rolls	High	73
Hamburger bun	Medium	61
Baguette	High	95
Pita bread (white)	Medium	57
Tortilla (wheat)	Low	30
BREAKFAST CEREALS		
All-Bran	Low	42
Oatmeal (not instant)	Low	49
Shredded wheat	Medium	69
Rice Krispies	High	82
Cornflakes	High	83
SNACKS AND SWEETS		
Cashews	Low	22

FOOD	RATING	GLYCEMIC INDEX
Peanuts	Low	14
Yogurt (low-fat)	Low	14
Ice cream (low-fat)	Low	50
Ice cream	Medium	61
Popcorn	Medium	55
Potato chips	Medium	57
Corn chips	High	74
Pretzels	High	81
Pop Tarts	High	70
Jelly beans	High	80
Life Savers	High	70
FRUITS		
Apples	Low	38
Bananas	Low	52
Cherries	Low	22
Grapefruit	Low	25
Plums	Low	39
Peaches	Low	42
Oranges	Low	44
Grapes	Low	46
Pears	Low	38
Pineapple	Medium	66
Strawberries	Low	40
Watermelon	High	72
VEGETABLES		
Asparagus	Low	15
Broccoli	Low	15

FOOD	RATING	GLYCEMIC INDEX
Carrots	Low	49
Cauliflower	Low	15
Celery	Low	15
Cucumber	Low	15
French fries	High	75
Peppers	Low	15
Parsnips	High	97
Eggplant	Low	15
Green beans	Low	15
Green peas	Low	48
Lettuce	Low	15
Potato, baked	High	85
Potato, new	Medium	57
Spinach	Low	15
Sweet potato	Low	54
Tomato	Low	15
Yam, boiled	Low	35
Zucchini	Low	15

The slower the foods you eat—and that means a low glycemic index—the longer you will feel full. If you change the composition of your meals and snacks, you can lower your glycemic index. The next chapter, Turn Up Your Metabolism, will show you how to combine your food and put your meals together to support easy digestion and high energy.

Detox Success Story
FREEDOM FROM PAIN

I have struggled with my weight for forty-five years, since adolescence. Because I had been raised on the standard American diet of the 1950s and '60s, loaded with dairy, meat, and refined sugars, things like constipation, excess weight, mood swings, and lack of energy were the norm. As a teen I tried Weight Watchers with little success; in my twenties, I switched to a high-fiber diet, eliminating sugar, and was able to normalize and maintain my weight at about 125, which suited my five-foot, three-inch frame quite well. I continued to eat lean meats and low-fat or nonfat dairy; I also used artificial sweeteners, processed oils, and salt extensively. I've always been what they call a social drinker. Since I've been single most of my life, I socialized a lot! I was a fairly serious caffeine junkie as well, using coffee in the morning and diet colas in the afternoon to keep my motor running. I never exercised. Add to all of this a two- to four-pack-a-day cigarette habit starting at age 14, and you can see how by age 30 I'd become a poster child for the slogan, "Live fast, die young, leave a pretty corpse."

I very nearly fulfilled that prophecy when two weeks before my thirty-seventh birthday, I had a stroke. I was paralyzed from the neck down on the right side for a month. After four weeks in tears and anger, asking "Why me?," I began to realize that the stroke was a wake-up call to take control of my health destiny. As I relearned the skills we all take for granted, like walking, writing, cooking, bathing, and tying my shoes, I vowed to embrace and value the life that hadn't yet been taken from me. I quit smoking, began exercising, and watched my diet in terms of sodium content, fats, and sugars. I did everything the doctors told me. Within six months I was able to return to my job as a legal secretary. I had stopped smoking and was at a reasonable weight, but I still consumed artificial sweeteners, heavily processed foods, and of course medications.

I continued to thrive, but decided it was time to take my weight from "reasonable" to "normal, healthy, and attractive." I adopted a vegan diet, which enabled me to lose weight sensibly without ever feeling deprived or hungry. I dropped from about 155 to a nice

130 pounds and managed to stay there . . . for a while. Even though I was vegan, the pounds crept back on. I was in my forties, with a slowing metabolism, and what was once a battle with my weight became an all-out war that appeared unwinnable.

In 2002, I developed Bell's palsy, a paralysis of the facial muscles that usually resolves itself within three months, six at the latest. Mine never did. My facial muscles required extensive electromuscular therapy to enable me to close one eye normally. I was left to contend with a drooping mouth, and worse yet, a persistent pain and itching deep in my inner ear.

By 2008, my weight was back up, this time to 168. I knew my life had to change, starting with leaving a nine-year relationship that wasn't working. Around that time, I heard one of my media heroes, Robin Quivers, describe the Martha's Vineyard Diet Detox, a new, vegan diet regimen she was trying, on the *Howard Stern Show*. I listened every day as Dr. Roni DeLuz shadowed Robin for a week at the radio station, describing the consumption of green drinks, fresh juices, and organic vegetable soups. I became excited about Robin's prospects for success and silently cheered for her every step of the way. Several months later, when it was clear that Robin's weight loss had been not only significant but lasting, I was convinced that this was the program for me!

It took me until January 2010 to get up the nerve to do the detox. After all, things like colonics and coffee enemas can seem a little daunting, and there was no way I could afford to spend a week at the Martha's Vineyard Holistic Retreat. Then there was the cost of the supplements, where to find them, selecting a colon therapist, and on and on. All of which, of course, were just mental stall tactics to avoid taking the bull by the horns and just doing it!

Once I started to focus on all the reasons I wanted and needed to do the detox—long-term weight control, improved health, and (hopefully) freedom from pain—the obstacles fell away, and I went for it. I started on the weekend to make the first two days as stress-free as possible. During that first twenty-one-day detox, I experienced a slight "healing crisis" around Day 5, in the form of head and body aches, dry mouth, incessant thirst, and complete lack of energy. I upped my intake of water and free soup, rode it out, and slept that night like a baby. By the end of the first week, I felt clearheaded, light, and pain-free, with no hunger issues whatsoever. After Day 5, I continued to feel that way for the duration of the detox. For the first time in years, I had no pain. When Day 22 rolled around, I actually dreaded the idea of having to prepare food again! I'd lost only seventeen pounds in twenty-one days. As I continued on the maintenance plan, I was able to get my weight down to 128 within six months—a total loss of forty pounds! I decided, right then and there, that I would detox annually from that point on.

The "new me" drew a steady stream of compliments and queries of "How did you do this?" For the first time in my life, buying and wearing clothes was pure joy, having gone from a size 16 to a size 6. I became a platinum blonde and decided to leave Atlanta and return to San Francisco. While I was orchestrating the move, I took a vacation to Florida to visit my mom and show off my new beach body. This was about six months after my first detox. I opted for a road trip and switched into full vacation mode. As I left Atlanta, I grabbed a fast-food breakfast burrito with everything but cheese, a cup of coffee, and some home fries. Midway to my mom's, I grabbed a mocha frappuccino for added caffeine to fuel my drive. That night at Mom's, I dove happily into a bottle of good California merlot. For four full days, I threw caution to the wind. On the fifth day, I awoke with a full-blown recurrence of Bell's palsy symptoms, including the return of that awful itching pain as well as a complete relapse of right-sided facial paralysis.

After another whirlwind round of neurologists, chiropractors, acupuncturists, and herbalists, I recovered reasonably well but not completely. It wasn't until my next detox, in January 2011, that I realized what the doctors couldn't and wouldn't: the "relapse" had been nothing more than my body's reaction to a sudden influx of toxins. About five days into detox number two, the pain subsided and I regained moderate function in my facial muscles. DUH! No more breakfast burritos or bingeing on coffee and wine for me.

My new mantra is "Detox annually." Just as I vowed never to binge on toxic food and drink again, I have now vowed never to skip a detox.

Suzy Vincent

CHAPTER 13

༄

TURN UP YOUR METABOLISM

Cheeseburgers with french fries; egg, bacon, and cheese on an English muffin; steak and potatoes; spaghetti and meatballs—these are classic meals in the standard American diet that are making us fatter and sicker. After eating one of these classics, you might feel gassy, bloated, dehydrated, or tired. These meals combine foods in a way that messes with your digestion. The main reason the composition of these meals leads to problems is that different food groups require different digestion times. Combining foods correctly allows your body to digest and utilize nutrients to the fullest extent. Following the rules of food combining enhances your digestion, producing more energy and helping you lose weight and keep it off. Once you start eating this way, "square meals" will become a thing of the past. You will realize that the way you have been taught to eat has compromised your digestive system, your attempts at weight loss, and your health.

Proteins need a highly acidic environment for digestion. Carbohydrates require an alkaline environment. If you eat a protein and a carbohydrate at the same time, you create a clash in your digestive system that causes indigestion, poor absorption of essential nutrients, and weight gain. The central principle of food combining is that meals be kept simple so that they can be digested properly by enzymes. Different foods, even foods in the same basic category, require unique enzymes. When you eat proteins like meat, fish, poultry, and eggs, your stomach secretes hydrochloric acid and the enzyme pepsin to break down the food in a highly acidic environment. When you eat bread, potatoes, or other starches, you secrete the enzyme ptyalin to create an alkaline condition. If you eat proteins and starches together, the enzymes neutralize each other, and digestion is inhibited.

Too many different foods in one meal confuse the body, which has difficulty producing all the necessary enzymes simultaneously. When food is poorly digested, it can become trapped in your digestive tract, where it putrefies. Your blood becomes more acidic, creating an environment in which disease-causing pathogens, yeasts, viruses, parasites, and cancer cells thrive. In addition, if your body cannot use the food, getting rid of it expends energy and overworks the organs of elimination. Since every food we eat is digested differently, it is essential to eat foods in the right combination for easy digestion and metabolism.

Foods require different amounts of time to be digested, so time has a role in food combining. What you want to avoid is a traffic jam in your digestive system. A rule of thumb is that denser foods are harder to digest and take longer to pass through. The following chart will give you a sense of how long it takes to digest the food you eat.

TIME FOR FOOD TO MOVE THROUGH THE STOMACH AND BE DIGESTED

FOOD	AVERAGE TRANSIT TIME	FULL DIGESTION
Water	0–10 minutes	10 minutes
Juice	15–30 minutes	15–30 minutes
Fruit	30–60 minutes	2–3 hours
Melons	15–30 minutes	up to 2 hours
Vegetables	2½ hours	up to 5 hours
Dense vegetable protein (nuts, seeds, avocados)	2–3 hours	12 hours

Protein fat (cheeses, milk, yogurt)	2–3 hours	12 hours
Beans	3–4 hours	12 hours
Starches	1–2 hours	5 hours
Cooked meat, fish, shellfish	3–4 hours	12 hours
Fats and oils	3–4 hours	12 hours
Any improperly combined meal	8 hours	24+ hours

By looking at how long it takes food to digest, you can also understand why meal timing is important. After you eat a grain-based meal, you should wait at least two to three hours before you eat protein. After a meal that contains protein, give yourself four hours to digest the meal. Remember to take your enzymes when you eat, and refrain from drinking during meals. The fluids will dilute your enzymes and slow down digestion.

Tossing and Turning

Do you find yourself counting sheep at night or watching reruns of infomercials? If so, the answer to your lost sleep may lie not in a pill but in some dietary tweaks. You probably already know that foods like chili, tomatoes, and peppermint can keep you awake by giving you acid indigestion. But did you know that combining protein and carbohydrates can keep you up as well? Here's how.

Say that it is 8:00 p.m. by the time you pick up your daughter after her basketball game. You run through the drive-through for a burger and fries—a deadly mix of protein, starch, and fat—but you still try to be mindful and choose not to supersize. You eat at eight-thirty, then go to bed at ten-thirty, needing to be fresh in the morning.

Even though you're ready to sleep, your body's still working overtime, trying to digest the food you have eaten. There is a clash of enzymes in your stomach that are trying to break down the difficult-to-digest dinner. Your stomach is gurgling. You may feel abdominal discomfort or heartburn.

You might start to worry about how tired you are going to be in the morning, start running tapes of conversations that took place during the day, or fret about all that is left on your to-do list.

Observing the rules of food combining and taking enzymes whenever you have a meal that requires chewing will help you avoid indigestion. If indigestion has routinely disturbed your sleep in the past, you should try eating your big meal and animal protein at lunch. Eating easy-to-digest foods at night—like soup, salad, whole grains, and whole-grain pasta—might help you to get a good night's sleep.

THE RULES OF FOOD COMBINING

After having completed the detox, your body is in gear to digest what you eat efficiently and to put the energy to good use. If you pay attention to combining your food in a way that allows your digestive system to work efficiently, it will fire up your metabolism and help you to lose weight and keep it off.

The rules of food combining might seem complicated at first, but they are very straightforward. If you follow these rules, you will save your body from processing incompatible food combinations that result in undigested food stagnating in your intestinal tract, leading to fermentation, putrefaction, an overgrowth of bacteria, and toxicity. To improve your digestion, follow these food-combining tips.

1. **Do not eat proteins and starches together.** Avoid eating simple carbohydrates and protein in the same meal. Bread, rice, potatoes, and cereals should not be mixed with fish, eggs, meat, dairy products, or tofu. This is the worst food combination there is. Your body requires an alkaline base to digest starches and an acid base to digest proteins. Digestion begins with the salivary glands producing the alkaline enzyme ptyalin when chewing begins. The enzyme begins to break down the starch, but the presence of the alkaline enzyme prevents the digestion of proteins in the stomach by pepsin and other acidic secretions. The meat putrefies in the digestive tract and bacteria attack the undigested meat, resulting in a heavy, bloated feeling and toxic waste.

Proteins and starches each combine well with green leafy vegetables and nonstarchy vegetables, but they do not work well together.

2. **Eat protein with vegetables only.**

3. **Eat starches like rice, bread, potatoes, pasta, and** foods made from flour **with vegetables only.**

4. **Fruits should be eaten alone or with other fruits, two hours before or after meals.** Fruits digest so quickly that by the time they reach your stomach they are already partially digested. If they are mixed with other foods, they will rot and ferment.

5. **Always eat melons on their own.** Melons digest more quickly than any other food. You should not eat melons with other food, including other fruits.

6. **Do not mix starch and sugar.** Those pastries and cookies may be tempting, but they stress your digestive system. When sugar and starches are combined in the mouth, the alkaline enzyme needed to digest starches, ptyalin, is stopped and starches remain undigested. Sugar ferments in the digestive tract and creates an acidic environment that further inhibits the digestion of starches.

7. **Avoid milk or drink it by itself.** Pasteurization destroys the natural enzymes in milk that make it digestible. Milk curdles when it reaches the stomach, coagulates with other foods, and prevents other foods from being digested. If you have to drink milk, drink raw milk or almond milk.

8. **Skip the sweet desserts.** Eating sweet, starchy desserts or sweet fruits after a meal will interrupt the digestion of carbohydrates or protein already in the stomach. Eating something sweet right after a meal essentially stops digestion. If you have to have something sweet, wait at least two hours after a meal.

It may not be possible to follow these rules to the letter, but if you make an attempt to follow these guidelines when you are planning your meals, your digestion will improve. Just following a few of these rules with healthy food choices will make you feel lighter and more energetic. The improvement in your metabolism will help to keep your weight down and flatten your stomach. Even more important, you will be reducing your toxic load.

The following chart is a quick reference to the rules of food combination.

FOOD COMBINING

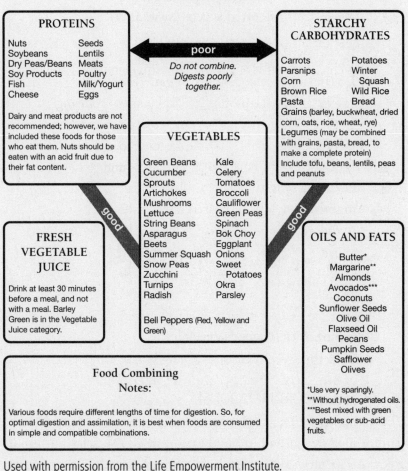

PROTEINS

Nuts   Seeds
Soybeans   Lentils
Dry Peas/Beans   Meats
Soy Products   Poultry
Fish   Milk/Yogurt
Cheese   Eggs

Dairy and meat products are not recommended; however, we have included these foods for those who eat them. Nuts should be eaten with an acid fruit due to their fat content.

poor
Do not combine. Digests poorly together.

STARCHY CARBOHYDRATES

Carrots   Potatoes
Parsnips   Winter
Corn   Squash
Brown Rice   Wild Rice
Pasta   Bread
Grains (barley, buckwheat, dried corn, oats, rice, wheat, rye)
Legumes (may be combined with grains, pasta, bread, to make a complete protein)
Include tofu, beans, lentils, peas and peanuts

VEGETABLES

Green Beans   Kale
Cucumber   Celery
Sprouts   Tomatoes
Artichokes   Broccoli
Mushrooms   Cauliflower
Lettuce   Green Peas
String Beans   Spinach
Asparagus   Bok Choy
Beets   Eggplant
Summer Squash   Onions
Snow Peas   Sweet
Zucchini   Potatoes
Turnips   Okra
Radish   Parsley

Bell Peppers (Red, Yellow and Green)

good

FRESH VEGETABLE JUICE

Drink at least 30 minutes before a meal, and not with a meal. Barley Green is in the Vegetable Juice category.

OILS AND FATS

Butter*
Margarine**
Almonds
Avocados***
Coconuts
Sunflower Seeds
Olive Oil
Flaxseed Oil
Pecans
Pumpkin Seeds
Safflower
Olives

*Use very sparingly.
**Without hydrogenated oils.
***Best mixed with green vegetables or sub-acid fruits.

Food Combining Notes:

Various foods require different lengths of time for digestion. So, for optimal digestion and assimilation, it is best when foods are consumed in simple and compatible combinations.

Used with permission from the Life Empowerment Institute.

Though we will be giving you two weeks of menus in Chapter 15, here are two days of meals that follow the food combining rules. As you experiment with constructing meals according to the guidelines, the rules will seem less confining because the possibilities are limitless.

Sample Menu #1

BREAKFAST
Hot water with lemon or green tea
Oatmeal with cinnamon, or a protein smoothie

LUNCH
Green salad with assorted vegetables and turkey

DINNER
Roast chicken with root vegetables and greens

Sample Menu #2

BREAKFAST
Toasted seven-grain bread with butter, or a spinach and
    mushroom omelet
Green tea

LUNCH
Vegetable soup with whole-grain bread, or whole-grain
    pasta with pesto

DINNER
Grilled fish with steamed vegetables

FOODS THAT BOOST METABOLISM

The only ways to change your metabolism permanently are to gain or lose weight and to build extra muscle. Muscles burn more calories than fat, making your body's engine run faster. Lean muscle makes your body a calorie-burning machine. Your eating schedule on Dr. Roni's Healthy Eating Plan also contributes to increasing your metabolism. When you eat large meals with hours before your next meal, your metabolism slows down between meals. Nourishing your body every few hours keeps your metabolism going so you burn more calories during the course of a day. By providing your body with dense nutrients at regular intervals, you will eat less at regular mealtimes. Certain foods increase metabolism and serve to help you stabilize the weight you have lost during the detox. Here are some foods that will speed up your metabolism.

Oatmeal: To jump-start your metabolism in the morning, start the day with a bowl of steel-cut oatmeal. A super food, oatmeal is rich in fat-soluble fiber, which takes a lot of calories to break down. Eating oatmeal can decrease cholesterol levels as well.

Grapefruit can reduce insulin levels. Lower insulin levels after eating can help your body process food more efficiently. With less insulin, you burn more calories and store less energy as fat.

Apples and pears: Studies have shown that these two fruits help boost metabolism and speed up weight loss. One study put two groups of women on identical diets, except that one group ate three small organic apples or pears a day. The group that ate the fruit lost more weight than the women who did not.

Hot peppers: Chemical compounds in spicy foods can kick the metabolism into a higher gear. Capsaicin gives peppers their heat. Eating a tablespoon of chopped red or green chile pepper can boost your metabolic rate temporarily. Spice up pasta dishes, chili, and stews with red pepper flakes. Capsaicin keeps the calorie burning elevated long after you have finished a meal.

Lean protein: The body burns up many more calories digesting protein than it uses on carbohydrates. The protein found in white meat chicken, turkey, other lean meats, fish, nuts, beans, and eggs takes a great deal of energy to break down. Protein is needed to build lean muscle mass, which burns more calories than fat.

Salmon and tuna: High levels of leptin are associated with slower metabolisms and with weight gain. Eating fish is a good way to lower leptin levels. The omega-3 fatty acids found in salmon and tuna cut leptin levels and help your body process foods more effectively. Omega-3 fatty acids are also found in anchovies, sardines, mackerel, and flax-seed oil.

Soup: Studies show that people who eat soup first consume less solid food for the rest of their meal. One study found that soup offered an appetite-reducing combination of liquids and solids that prevented the intake of excess foods, speeding up the metabolism for fat burning.

Greek-style yogurt: Yogurt is packed with calcium and protein. It gives you lots of energy and helps in the building of lean muscle mass. Yogurt with live cultures helps to regulate your digestive tract by contributing microflora.

Broccoli: Rich in calcium and vitamin C, broccoli helps you to burn calories faster. Calcium activates your metabolism while vitamin C helps you to absorb more calcium.

Almonds: Though high in calories, almonds are packed with essential fatty acids that boost your metabolism.

Green tea: The caffeine in green tea accelerates your heart rate and speeds up your metabolism. Another chemical present in green tea, epigallocatechin gallate (EGCG), stimulates the nervous system and helps to burn calories at a faster rate.

Black coffee: The shot of caffeine you get from coffee increases energy and concentration. If consumed in moderation, coffee can cause a short-term boost in your metabolic rate.

* * *

You now know the principles that form the foundation of Dr. Roni's Healthy Eating Plan. You are equipped to make informed choices about the best way to nourish your body. This part of the book is designed for you to keep handy and to use as a quick reference to support you in making healthy food choices. It is important for you to understand what makes this plan work. When you are familiar with the mechanics of metabolism, you are more highly motivated to keep your body well fueled. If you do your best to make eating according to these guidelines a way of life, you will lock in all the improvements you made during the detox and will enjoy continued good health.

No matter how determined you are to eat well, no one is perfect. You might stray beyond the 25 percent. Do not be too hard on yourself if you do. You can get right back to a healthy routine and recuperate from backsliding. In addition to occasional lapses, you still live in a toxic world and will continue to be exposed to harmful chemicals that are beyond your control. That is why you have to consider the 1 Pound a Day Diet Detox an annual event. The next chapter will explain how to know when you need to detox and give you two-day and seven-day detoxes for tune-ups.

Detox Success Story
I FELT LIKE A TEENAGER

In January of every year, my church does a fast. We are strongly encouraged to take part. Every year my husband and I decide to do it. In January 2011 I made the decision that my husband and I were going to do the detox that I originally heard about on Steve Harvey's show—the Martha's Vineyard Diet Detox. I told my husband, who said it sounded like a great plan. Over the years, I have dieted more times that I can count, and nothing has really stuck with me. This time around I wanted a life change.

I was at my heaviest, about 240 pounds. My bra size was the largest it has ever been—42F. I was disgusted with myself and knew I had to change. I had the worst heartburn. Everything I ate gave me heartburn. The worst gas ever! I was embarrassed even around my own husband. My eczema and allergies were at their worst.

When I heard Steve Harvey talking about the detox on the radio, I got the book. I couldn't put it down. I was amazed by everything I read. I felt like a big ball of toxins ready to explode. This was a wake-up call to get my life back together and get control of myself. During the holidays, I cleaned out my fridge and got things together. I researched all the whole food stores around me. I found that the closest place for me to get a colonic was an hour away, and the procedure was expensive. But I was determined!

The detox changed my life forever. I lost the 21 pounds in 21 days. In the weeks that followed I continued to lose weight, because even after the detox I didn't introduce meat or soda back into my diet for about another month. I stopped eating pork for six months. Yes, it was hard, probably the hardest thing I had ever done. But afterward, I felt the best that I had ever felt in my adult years. I was thirty-one years old and I felt like a teenager. In total, I lost thirty-one pounds.

Janicca S. Covington

CHAPTER 14

⌒

YOUR BODY DESERVES A FIVE-STAR VACATION AND REGULAR GETAWAYS

You do not do the 1 Pound a Day Diet Detox once in your life and then forget about it. All the systems in your body work hard and deserve a sabbatical for restoration at least once a year. Doing the full detox annually is the best way to stay slim, boost your energy, and sustain your radiant health. Detoxing is the best antiaging technique you can find. Plan to set a month aside each year to cleanse your body of toxins that have accumulated and to heal any damage these poisons may have done. You have already experienced how light you are physically, mentally, and spiritually after completing the thirty-day detox. In the course of the year, you may feel some of the benefits fading, depending on how well you follow Dr. Roni's Healthy Eating Plan and what is happening in your life. Life-changing events and everyday stress can take their toll on your equilibrium in body, mind, and spirit. When you feel your sense of well-being slipping, you will know it is time to stop the slide. This chapter gives you the techniques to make the corrections.

You might find yourself making bad food choices. That bloated, heavy sensation returns. You could sense an emotional shift as toxins build up. You might feel deflated in spirit. Your optimism and joy turn down a few notches as your irritability and anger rise. Life's stresses start getting to you. You can feel your resilience draining.

You might have trouble sleeping, start craving junk food, or not be hungry at all. Brain fog can take over.

You will come to read your body and know when your toxic load is beginning to affect your well-being. Over time, you will be familiar with the rhythm of your body and know when it needs the break that the 1 Pound a Day Diet Detox will give you. You take time off for a vacation every year—even if it is just catching up on sleep and getting your life in order. You can give your body a five-star, luxurious retreat by doing the thirty-day detox annually. It will restore your health, extend your life, and make you look as if you have been pampered at a posh spa.

> I have not been perfect with my diet, but if I find myself straying too far, I just juice for an entire day, and that gets me back on track. I truly believe that the detox has reset my metabolism, and that is why I haven't gained the weight back.
>
> Susan Keane

You might want to pick a particular time of year for your yearly detox. Many veteran detoxers like to start the year clean and detox right after the holidays—a new you for the New Year. You might prefer to detox before Memorial Day so that your body is in top shape for the summer. Maybe you are still in the back-to-school frame of mind and want to get your act together after the summer ends. You may decide you do not want to commit to detoxing at a particular time each year and would rather respond to the way you are feeling. Whatever works for you is the right time, as long as you do it.

As you repeat the detox, it will become easier each time. You know what to expect, and you have the logistics of the detox down. You have your favorite juice combinations and soups. The time flies faster with each successive detox, and the results get deeper.

CORRECTIONS FOR BACKSLIDING

If your off-the-plan eating is moving up from 25 percent and you feel as if you are going off the rails, do not lose heart. It is easy to regress. If you are very busy or under stress, you might find yourself reaching for convenience foods to save time, or craving comfort foods that you thought were a thing of the past. You have managed to live without junky processed foods, but they do have an insidious way of slipping back into your diet. No matter how motivated you are right now, falling back into bad habits can be easier than you think. But you have a way to remedy the situation. If you find your weight inching up, it is time to do something about it. You can do an abbreviated version of the 1 Pound a Day Diet Detox, lose the weight you have put back on, and reinforce the good habits you are trying to form.

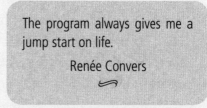

> The program always gives me a jump start on life.
>
> Renée Convers

Some detoxers advise weighing in every day. A two-pound weight gain motivates them to do a single day of fresh juice and soup, or a vegetarian day. That can do the trick. The more weight that you allow to creep back on and the more unhealthy eating you do, the longer you will have to spend on the detox regimen to get back to where you started from.

Two-Day Detox

Some of the happiest detoxers build two days of detoxing into every week; this allows them to keep the healing and weight-loss momentum going. Some do this on Monday and Tuesday to compensate for more relaxed eating at home and at social events during the weekend. Some, who are very busy during the week with work and family schedules, feel they can manage what they eat more easily during the weekend, when they have more time to juice and make soup.

Other detoxers are not as consistent. They may chose to do two days of detoxing now and then when they feel out of sorts, have been under a lot of stress, or suddenly find themselves craving sweets and junk food. This quick tune-up can restore you if you have not let go too long or too far. Just dive right in and follow the daily schedule for the 1 Pound a Day Diet Detox on page 232 for two days.

Support your detox with a cleansing bath and dry skin brushing. If you cannot get a colonic, try to have a coffee enema.

To transition from the Two-Day Detox, continue to drink green juice, cleansing soup, and broth and take all of your supplements for a day. Add healthy food without chemicals and toxins—maybe a salad for lunch or brown rice in your soup. It is important that you continue to drink six to eight ounces of water between meals, totaling forty-eight to sixty-four ounces each day. You can return to Dr. Roni's Healthy Eating Plan the following day.

Seven-Day Detox

We recommend that you do a seven-day detox each season you are not doing the full detox. These regular tune-ups will keep your body functioning at optimal levels, which will protect you from disease. You may feel the need for a bigger correction anytime. If you are coming down from your detox high, you might not want to wait until your symptoms get worse. Maybe you have been traveling and were too tempted by the local cuisine to be moderate in your eating. Or you could have had a deadline for a business project that became your top priority. Or your weight has been slowly moving up. A week on the 1 Pound a Day Diet Detox will get you back on track.

It should not be difficult to find seven days to concentrate on detoxing. Consider it a getaway from the distractions and demands that made you lose sight of your goal. Think about what particular guidelines from Dr. Roni's Healthy Eating Plan were causing you trouble. Did you forget to take your supplements? Were you drinking enough water? Were you craving junk food? What time of day were you most likely to go off the plan? Were your cravings connected to events or emotions? By examining your behavior, you can get insights into your relationship with food. This week will revitalize you and reanimate your resolve to follow Dr. Roni's Healthy Eating Plan.

Take the time to pamper yourself during the week as if you were at a luxurious celebrity-filled spa. Have a detox bath, a body wrap, a lymphatic massage, a colonic, or all of the above. Make this quick detox fun.

FOUR DAYS BACK TO THE FULL HEALTHY EATING PLAN (PLUS ONE)

Transition Day 1

Continue with your juice, cleansing soups, broth, supplements, and distilled water. Add a cup of fruit, as long as you eat it two hours before or after a meal. For lunch, have a small raw vegetable salad or cooked vegetable with no dressing, oil, or vinegar. You can squeeze fresh lemon juice on the salad or vegetable.

Transition Day 2

Continue to eat the foods and supplements you ate on Day 1. Add a serving of a whole-grain cereal like oatmeal, whole-grain bread, millet, quinoa, or brown rice.

Transition Day 3

Repeat Day 2, adding a protein smoothie and one teaspoon of an essential fatty acid liquid or flaxseed oil. You can add the oil or EFA liquid to a salad, a vegetable dish, or your smoothie.

Transition Day 4

Repeat Day 3, adding other proteins, including eggs, soy, nuts, legumes, and beans. You can have three to four ounces of boiled, broiled, grilled, or baked fish and chicken.

Transition Day 5

If you wish, you may add red meat and resume Dr. Roni's Healthy Eating Plan.

* * *

Now you know how to give your body a five-star vacation or to have a quick, restorative getaway to reverse the effects of backsliding. You will be able to control your weight. You can wave goodbye to those pounds and inches that you have lost forever. You can give your old clothes away, confident that if things get out of hand you have a simple plan to do what you have to do to stay in top shape. You will look forward to the clarity and happiness that detoxing delivers, believe us. You have the ability to transform your life. Go for it!

The final chapter will prove to you that healthy eating can be even more scrumptious than what you used to eat. You will find two weeks of mouthwatering meals on Dr. Roni's Healthy Eating Plan along with delectable recipes from Dr. Roni's kitchen.

> This is my second tour of duty on the detox, and this is my ninth day. I weighed in today—said goodbye to the 300s. Yup, for the first time since my eleven-year-old son was born, I am under the 300-pound mark!
>
> I'm not looking back! I'm getting ready for my close-up. Next year by this time, you can't tell me nuthin'! No stopping us now—we are on the move. I am proud of myself.
>
> Barbara Wilson

~

DR. RONI'S HEALTHY EATING PLAN: MEAL PLANS AND RECIPES FOR THE REST OF YOUR LIFE

Carnivore, vegan, piscatarian; Italian, French, Thai, Mexican, Middle Eastern, or Southern food fan—there are so many styles of eating today and such a diversity of cuisines. On Dr. Roni's Healthy Eating Plan, you do not have to give up eating the foods and flavors you love. You can apply the principles of the plan to whatever way you like to eat.

You have learned a lot about good nutrition in the preceding chapters. You might be feeling a bit overwhelmed. Our goal in this section has been to give you the reasons why these guidelines are so important for your continued good health. In this chapter, we want to put it all together to show you how these rules apply to your daily eating by providing you with meal plans to get you off to a great start and recipes you and your family will enjoy.

The rules might be a big departure from the way you used to eat. You have wiped the slate clean and are ready to start over. You have made the transition from what you ate on the 1 Pound a Day Diet Detox over a nine-day period. You are ready to make food choices that will keep your vitality high, your new weight stable, and your health robust.

To get you accustomed to your new way of eating, Dr. Roni has worked up two full weeks of meal plans. Remember to take enzymes whenever you chew. Drink a glass of filtered or spring water on odd hours to stay fully hydrated. If you are eating fruit as a snack, wait at least two hours after a meal to do so.

Dr. Roni's Rules for Healthy Eating

The ten rules for healthy eating distill the nutritional information found in the previous chapters. If you follow these rules 75 percent of the time, you will maintain your weight loss, high energy, and good spirits.

1. Eat only natural foods.
2. Eat only whole foods.
3. Eat mostly live foods—75 percent of your diet.
4. Eat only toxin-free foods.
5. Eat only sugar-free foods.
6. Eat foods high in complex carbohydrates.
7. Eat foods high in essential fatty acids, like nuts and flaxseeds.
8. Do not eat table salt.
9. Eat meals that are combined correctly.
10. Limit animal protein to three times a week.

Two-Week Meal Plan

DAY 1

Awake: Hot water with lemon, or green tea, or 1 ounce of antioxidant berry drink

Breakfast: Steel-cut oatmeal with slivered almonds and cinnamon with almond milk

Midmorning Snack: Green drink

Lunch: Mixed vegetable salad

Afternoon Snack: Carrot sticks with cashew butter

Dinner: Citrus Salmon with Greens (page 259)

Snack: Small bowl of berries

DAY 2

Awake: Hot water with lemon, or green tea, or 1 ounce of antioxidant berry drink

Breakfast: Peppermint Freeze Smoothie (page 268)

Midmorning Snack: Green juice

Lunch: Virtuous Vegetable Soup (page 252)

Afternoon Snack: ¼ cup raw almonds

Dinner: Quinoa pasta with broccoli

Snack: ½ cup Greek-style yogurt

DAY 3

Awake: Hot water with lemon, or green tea, or 1 ounce of antioxidant berry drink

Breakfast: Steamed kale with soft-boiled eggs

Midmorning Snack: Green juice

Lunch: Veggie burger with whole-grain bread

Afternoon Snack: Protein smoothie with cashew butter

Dinner: Red Beans and Rice Casserole (page 257)

Snack: ½ grapefruit

DAY 4

Awake: Hot water with lemon, or green tea, or 1 ounce of antioxidant berry drink

Breakfast: Vanilla nut protein smoothie

Midmorning Snack: Green drink

Lunch: Mixed vegetable salad

Afternoon Snack: ¼ cup sunflower seeds

Dinner: Vegetarian Chili (page 250)

Snack: Small bowl of cut-up melon

DAY 5

Awake: Hot water with lemon, or green tea, or 1 ounce of antioxidant berry drink

Breakfast: Millet porridge

Midmorning Snack: Green juice

Lunch: Whole-grain bread with sprouts, tomato, and cucumbers

Afternoon Snack: 1 cup cut-up melon

Dinner: Curried Chicken Sausage Casserole (page 261)

Snack: 6 ounces kale chips

DAY 6

Awake: Hot water with lemon, or green tea, or 1 ounce of antioxidant berry drink

Breakfast: Omelet with vegetables

Midmorning Snack: Green juice

Lunch: Spiced steamed veggies over brown rice

Afternoon Snack: 1 cup cut-up watermelon

Dinner: Spicy Bean Party Soup (page 253)

Snack: ¼ cup cashews

DAY 7

Awake: Hot water with lemon, or green tea, or 1 ounce of antioxidant berry drink

Breakfast: "Nuts for You" Cereal (page 238) with almond milk

Midmorning Snack: Green juice

Lunch: Raw spinach and avocado soup

Afternoon Snack: 1 cup berries

Dinner: Lime Veggie Pasta (page 261)

Snack: Cucumber slices with ¼ cup Greek-style yogurt

DAY 8

Awake: Hot water with lemon, or green tea, or 1 ounce of antioxidant berry drink

Breakfast: Scrambled eggs with onion, tomato, and cilantro

Midmorning Snack: Green drink

Lunch: Grilled Veggie Wrap (page 247)

Afternoon Snack: Celery sticks with almond butter

Dinner: Red Beans and Rice Casserole (page 257)

Snack: Orange Creamsicle Smoothie (page 266)

DAY 9

Awake: Hot water with lemon, or green tea, or 1 ounce of antioxidant berry drink

Breakfast: Banana and Almond Protein Shake (page 237)
Midmorning Snack: Green juice
Lunch: Carrot-Zucchini Stir-Fry (page 250)
Afternoon Snack: ¼ cup raw almonds
Dinner: Virtuous Vegetable Soup (page 252)
Snack: ¼ cup hummus with celery sticks

DAY 10
Awake: Hot water with lemon, or green tea, or 1 ounce of antioxidant berry drink
Breakfast: Poached eggs with asparagus
Midmorning Snack: Green juice
Lunch: Fresh mushroom soup
Afternoon Snack: Hummus and carrots
Dinner: Orange Chicken with Snow Peas and Asparagus (page 262)
Snack: Baked sweet potato chips

DAY 11
Awake: Hot water with lemon, or green tea, or 1 ounce of antioxidant berry drink
Breakfast: Protein smoothie
Midmorning Snack: Green drink
Lunch: Stir-fry vegetables with onion rings
Afternoon Snack: ¼ cup sunflower seeds
Dinner: Grilled sesame tuna
Snack: Sliced apple

DAY 12
Awake: Hot water with lemon, or green tea, or 1 ounce of antioxidant berry drink
Breakfast: Brown rice cereal with cinnamon and nutmeg
Midmorning Snack: Green juice
Lunch: Creamy Nutmeg Broccoli Soup (page 255)
Afternoon Snack: 1 cup cut-up melon

Dinner: Cajun tilapia with green beans

Snack: Chocolate Banana Split Smoothie (page 267)

DAY 13

Awake: Hot water with lemon, or green tea, or 1 ounce of antioxidant berry drink

Breakfast: Poached eggs with asparagus

Midmorning Snack: Green juice

Lunch: Steamed vegetables over barley

Afternoon Snack: Chocolate-coconut protein smoothie

Dinner: Herb Flatbread Pizza (page 249)

Snack: Mocha Shaker (page 267)

DAY 14

Awake: Hot water with lemon, or green tea, or 1 ounce of antioxidant berry drink

Breakfast: Whole-grain toast with sliced tomatoes and basil

Midmorning Snack: Green juice

Lunch: Veggie burger on whole-grain roll

Afternoon Snack: Mocha Shaker (page 267)

Dinner: Pasta with pesto sauce and veggies

Snack: 4 or 5 asparagus spears with tahini

FROM DR. RONI'S KITCHEN

Clean food does not have to be boring or bland. Forget any preconceptions you might have about "health food." As you will see in the recipes that follow, eating right does not mean sacrificing flavor and enjoyment. These easy-to-make dishes will keep you satisfied and well-nourished at the same time. You will probably be eating a greater variety of food than you have in the past. This food is so delicious that you will win over your family and friends when you serve them meals made from these recipes. The combination of observing your transformation and tasting this delicious food will make them converts to your new way of life.

Satisfying a Sweet Tooth

Do you have a taste for something sweet, love fruit-flavored soda, or get a kick out of carbonation? If so, try this healthy tip. Carry matchbook-size packets of Emergen-C (or a similar product that does not contain sugar) in your wallet or purse in orange, raspberry, lemon-lime, açai berry, or the fruit flavor of your choice. Whether you're at your desk or a restaurant, drop a packet into some plain water or seltzer. Within moments you'll be drinking a delicious fruity yet nontoxic beverage whose high dose of vitamin C also delivers an energy boost.

Another option is to use flavored stevia in water or club soda. It comes in many flavors, including vanilla cream, berry, Valencia orange, root beer, cinnamon, chocolate, chocolate raspberry, and English toffee. You will never miss the calorie-packed sodas or toxic diet sodas.

Breakfast Foods

BANANA AND ALMOND PROTEIN SHAKE

2 servings

3 to 5 ice cubes
12 to 16 raw almonds
2 scoops vanilla protein powder
1 cup almond milk
10 drops organic banana extract
5 drops organic rum extract
Pinch of ground cinnamon (optional)
Stevia

Combine the ice, almonds, protein powder, almond milk, extracts, and cinnamon, if using, in a blender. Blend until drinkable. Stir in stevia to taste and enjoy.

"NUTS FOR YOU" CEREAL

2 servings

¼ pound unsalted blanched almonds
¼ pound shelled walnuts
¼ pound shelled pecans
¼ pound unsalted hulled pumpkin seeds
2 cups or more rice milk (preferably Rice Dream), or almond or
    hemp milk
Stevia

1. Combine the almonds, walnuts, pecans, and pumpkin seeds in a food processor and pulse until the pieces are about ¼ inch.

2. Transfer the nuts to two bowls. Pour in the milk and sprinkle with stevia to taste. Let sit for a few minutes if you want the nuts to soften up.

CAULIFLOWER-EGG STIR-FRY

2 servings

2 tablespoons coconut oil
1 cup chopped cauliflower florets
¼ cup finely chopped onion
1 tablespoon very finely chopped garlic
1 teaspoon no-salt vegetable seasoning
Pinch of cayenne pepper
2 eggs, beaten

1. Heat the oil in a skillet over medium heat. Add the cauliflower, onion, and garlic and cook, stirring, until the onion begins to color.

2. Add the seasoning and cayenne and continue to cook and stir until the onion is soft and golden.

3. Reduce the heat to low and pour in the eggs. Stir from time to time for a scramble, or let cook undisturbed for an omelet. Cook until the eggs are done to your liking.

CURRIED EGGS, ZUCCHINI, AND SWEET PEAS

2 servings

½ cup finely chopped zucchini
½ cup organic frozen peas, thawed
1 teaspoon curry powder
½ teaspoon no-salt vegetable seasoning
Pinch of ground turmeric
Pinch of cayenne pepper
2 tablespoons coconut oil
2 eggs, beaten
4 to 6 large lettuce leaves

1. Bring a medium pot of water to a boil. Add the zucchini and peas and cook until crisp-tender, 2 to 3 minutes. Drain the vegetables in a colander in the sink and discard the water.

2. Combine the curry powder, seasoning, turmeric, and cayenne in a very small bowl.

3. Heat the oil in a medium skillet over medium heat. Stir in the spices. Add the zucchini and peas and stir until they are coated with the spices and oil. Cook, stirring from time to time, until the zucchini is lightly browned.

4. Reduce the heat to low and pour in the eggs. Stir from time to time for a scramble, or let cook undisturbed for an omelet. Cook until the eggs are done to your liking.

5. Place the lettuce on two plates. Top with the eggs and vegetables and serve.

Salad Dressings

Salads are a great way to increase your vegetable intake. There is nothing like a crunchy, fresh salad as a side dish or a main course. Chop up any raw vegetables and toss them with greens. You can add chicken, seafood, cooked grains, or beans for a dose of additional protein. If salad has always meant iceberg lettuce to you, branch out. Other lettuces are more nutritious. Baby spinach, arugula, spring mixes, romaine, and red leaf lettuce are all delicious and packed with phytonutrients. Add nuts for crunch and additional nutrients.

Here are some flavorful salad dressings you will love.

ITALIAN MUSTARD DRESSING

2 to 3 servings

¼ cup cider vinegar
2 tablespoons Dijon mustard
2 tablespoons very finely chopped fresh herbs, such as basil, oregano, chives, and/or thyme
2 garlic cloves, peeled and very finely chopped
Pinch of cayenne pepper
¼ cup olive oil

Combine the vinegar, mustard, herbs, garlic, and cayenne in a jar. Cover tightly and shake well. Add the oil and shake well until combined. Refrigerate any leftovers and use within 2 days.

ONION-GARLIC DRESSING

2 to 3 servings

¼ cup sour cream
¼ cup almond milk
2 tablespoons very finely chopped fresh parsley
1 tablespoon fresh lemon juice
2 teaspoons very finely chopped onion
1 large garlic clove, peeled and very finely chopped

Combine all the ingredients in a jar. Cover tightly and shake well until combined. Refrigerate any leftovers and use within 2 days.

CUCUMBER-ONION DRESSING

2 to 3 servings

¼ cup red wine vinegar
½ teaspoon sesame oil
2 tablespoons finely chopped red onion
2 tablespoons finely chopped cucumber
¼ teaspoon fresh minced garlic
¼ teaspoon no-salt vegetable seasoning
Pinch of dried basil
Pinch of cayenne pepper

Combine all the ingredients in a blender and puree until smooth. Chill before serving. Refrigerate any leftovers and use within 2 days.

GREEN BEAN DRESSING

2 to 3 servings

½ cup chopped raw green beans
¼ cup fresh lemon juice
¼ cup unflavored rice vinegar
Pinch of garlic powder
Pinch of cayenne pepper

Combine all the ingredients in a blender and puree until smooth. Chill before serving. This dressing will change color if stored, so try to use it all when fresh.

ITALIAN NATURALLY DRESSING

2 to 3 servings

½ cup balsamic vinegar
1 tablespoon flaxseed oil
1 tablespoon no-salt vegetable seasoning
1½ teaspoons finely chopped garlic
Pinch of dried basil
Pinch of dried oregano
Pinch of dried parsley
Pinch of cayenne pepper

Combine all the ingredients in a blender and puree until smooth. Chill before serving. Refrigerate any leftovers and use within 2 days.

SPICY MUSTARD DRESSING

2 to 3 servings

1 cup nonfat plain yogurt
2 tablespoons unflavored rice vinegar
2 teaspoons organic dry mustard
¼ teaspoon Bragg Liquid Aminos
Pinch of stevia

Combine all the ingredients in a blender and puree until smooth. Chill before serving. Refrigerate any leftovers and use within 2 days.

CAESAR GREEK DRESSING

2 to 3 servings

¼ cup Greek-style yogurt
¼ cup unflavored rice vinegar
4 kalamata olives, pitted and very finely chopped
½ teaspoon dried oregano
½ teaspoon dried thyme
½ teaspoon dried basil
½ teaspoon dried marjoram

1. Combine the yogurt, vinegar, and olives in a bowl and whisk to combine. Stir in the oregano, thyme, basil, and marjoram. Chill before serving. Refrigerate any leftovers and use within 2 days.

BALSAMIC BRAGG DRESSING

2 to 3 servings

2 carrots, peeled and chopped
½ cup Bragg Liquid Aminos
¼ cup balsamic vinegar or white balsamic vinegar
2 tablespoons flaxseed oil

Put the carrots in a food processor and chop as fine as possible. Add the liquid aminos, vinegar, and oil and process until well blended. Chill before serving. Refrigerate any leftovers and use within 2 days.

SWEET-AND-SOUR CARROT DRESSING

2 to 3 servings

1 small tomato
2 small carrots, peeled
¼ cup red wine vinegar
1 teaspoon fresh lemon juice
2 teaspoons stevia

1. Cut the tomato in half and squeeze out the seeds. Using a grater, grate the tomato flesh into a bowl.

2. Juice the carrots. Add the carrot juice, vinegar, lemon juice, and stevia to the tomato and stir to combine. Chill before serving. This dressing is best used fresh.

GINGER-SESAME DRESSING

2 to 3 servings

¼ cup fresh lemon juice
2 tablespoons cider vinegar
2 tablespoons sesame oil
1 teaspoon very finely chopped peeled fresh ginger
1 teaspoon stevia

Combine all the ingredients in a jar. Cover tightly and shake well until combined. Refrigerate any leftovers and use within 2 days.

AVOCADO CREAM DRESSING

2 to 3 servings

½ cup fresh lemon juice
Flesh of ½ avocado
¼ cup Tofutti (soy-based sour cream substitute)
1 teaspoon no-salt vegetable seasoning
Pinch of cayenne pepper

Combine all the ingredients in a blender and puree until smooth. Chill before serving. This dressing is best used fresh.

HOMEMADE MAYONNAISE

2 to 3 servings

1 whole egg
1 egg yolk
1 teaspoon fresh lemon juice
1 teaspoon Dijon mustard
Pinch of fine sea salt
2 tablespoons liquid coconut oil
1 teaspoon olive oil

1. Combine the egg, egg yolk, lemon juice, mustard, and salt in a blender. Blend on high speed until the mixture becomes creamy, about 30 seconds.

2. With the blender going, drizzle in the coconut oil very slowly, a few drops at a time. When that is all added, blend in the olive oil.

3. Transfer the mayonnaise to a glass jar, cover, and refrigerate until thickened. Keep refrigerated.

Lunches and Snacks

DEVILED EGGS SNACK

6 servings (2 halves each)

6 eggs
2 tablespoons Homemade Mayonnaise (see above) or store-
    bought organic mayonnaise
1 teaspoon cider vinegar
½ teaspoon Bragg Liquid Aminos
½ teaspoon Dijon mustard
¼ teaspoon stevia

Pinch of cayenne pepper
No-salt vegetable seasoning

1. Put the eggs in a pot and add water to cover by about 2 inches. Place over high heat and bring to a boil. Turn off the heat, cover the pot, and let sit for about 15 minutes.

2. Drain off the water and put the pot in the sink. Lightly crack the shells by knocking the eggs on the bottom of the pot. Run cold water over the eggs until they are cool. Peel and set aside to cool completely.

3. Combine the mayonnaise, vinegar, liquid aminos, mustard, stevia, and cayenne in a medium bowl. Cut the eggs in half lengthwise and add the yolks to the mayonnaise. Mash with a fork until smooth, thick, and well blended. Spoon the filling into the whites. Make a pattern on the top with a fork, if you like. Top each half with a pinch of seasoning.

4. Serve immediately, or chill before serving.

GRILLED VEGGIE WRAP
If you make these on a Sunday, you will have lunch for several days—that is, if there are any wraps left!

4 to 8 servings

1 small red onion, peeled, cut in half lengthwise, and sliced
    into half-moons
2 medium zucchini, cut lengthwise into ¼-inch slices (you'll
    need 12 slices)
2 small yellow squash, cut lengthwise into ¼-inch slices (you'll
    need 8 slices)
Olive oil
No-salt vegetable seasoning
Cayenne pepper

4 whole wheat wraps

1 cup hummus (preferably homemade, but store-bought is
   okay)

¼ cup toasted pine nuts

2 lightly packed cups baby spinach leaves

¼ cup chopped fresh mint leaves

1. Preheat the grill to medium or heat the grill pan over
medium heat. If using the grill, soak wooden skewers in water
while it's heating.

2. Lay out the onion, zucchini, and squash slices on a cookie
sheet. Run a skewer through each onion slice to hold it
together while grilling. Very lightly brush the vegetables with
oil and sprinkle lightly with seasoning and cayenne. Flip the
slices and brush and sprinkle the other side.

3. Grill the vegetables until tender and lightly browned,
flipping once, about 4 minutes per side. If using a grill pan, you
may have to work in batches.

4. Spread each wrap with ¼ cup of the hummus. Sprinkle
each with 1 tablespoon of the pine nuts. Top each with 3 slices
of zucchini, 2 slices of squash, ½ cup of the spinach, a few
onion slices, and 1 tablespoon of the mint. Roll up and cut in
half on a diagonal.

HERB FLATBREAD PIZZA

This is a healthy pizza substitute. Feel free to improvise. There are endless combinations of ingredients you can put on top of a pizza. Try artichoke hearts, cherry tomatoes, and pine nuts, or asparagus, shaved Brussels sprouts, and sliced almonds.

4 servings

Olive oil
1 large onion, peeled and sliced thin
1 medium to large whole wheat flatbread
¾ cup shredded soy-based cheddar cheese substitute
Florets from 1 small head broccoli, chopped into small pieces
1 teaspoon dried Italian herb seasoning
No-salt vegetable seasoning
Leaves from 3 rosemary sprigs, chopped
6 fresh basil leaves

Preheat the oven to 400°F.

1. While the oven is heating, put 1½ teaspoons olive oil in a large skillet and place over medium-high heat. When the oil is hot, add the onion. Stir just to separate the slices, then cook undisturbed for about 5 minutes, until the onion starts to color. Reduce the heat to medium-low and cook for 15 to 20 minutes, until the onion is deeply golden and caramelized. Stir from time to time to prevent the onion from sticking to the pan. Remove the pan from the heat.

2. Brush a cookie sheet very lightly with oil. Place the flatbread on the sheet and top with the onion, spreading it evenly. Sprinkle the cheese over the onion. Distribute the broccoli over the cheese. Sprinkle with the Italian seasoning and vegetable seasoning.

3. Bake for 18 minutes, or until the cheese is melted and light brown.

4. Remove from the oven and sprinkle with the rosemary and basil while still hot. Let cool for 5 minutes to allow ingredients to set. Slice and serve.

CARROT-ZUCCHINI STIR-FRY

4 servings

2 teaspoons coconut oil
4 carrots, peeled and cut into matchsticks
2 zucchini, trimmed and cut into matchsticks
2 tablespoons chopped fresh basil

1. Heat the oil in a large skillet over medium-high heat. When hot, add the carrots and zucchini. Stir for about 3 minutes, until crisp-tender.

2. Remove from the heat, sprinkle with the basil, and serve immediately.

Soups and Stews

VEGETARIAN CHILI

Nothing like a bowl of chili to fill you up on a cold day. This chili is so delicious you will not even miss the meat.

To add the texture of meat to a meatless chili, use tofu that was previously frozen. Freezing tofu alters its texture and makes it chewy like meat. After thawing the block of tofu, press it gently to remove excess water, then crumble.

4 servings

1½ tablespoons coconut oil
2 celery stalks, finely chopped
1 large onion, peeled and finely chopped

1 cup chopped green beans
1 pound firm organic tofu, crumbled
6 garlic cloves, peeled and very finely chopped
1 teaspoon cayenne pepper
6 fresh tomatoes, chopped
¼ cup water
2 cups cooked kidney beans (see page 258, or use organic
    beans in BPA-free cans), drained
¼ cup Bragg Liquid Aminos
½ cup chopped fresh parsley
Cooked brown rice, to serve

1. Heat the oil in a deep skillet or large pot over medium heat. Add the celery, onion, and green beans and cook for 3 minutes, stirring from time to time.

2. Add the tofu, garlic, and cayenne pepper. Cook for 5 minutes more.

3. Combine the tomatoes and water in a blender or food processor and puree. Add to the vegetables along with the kidney beans and liquid aminos. Cover and simmer for about 15 minutes, until the vegetables are cooked through and the flavors blended.

4. Remove from the heat and mix in the parsley to finish. Serve over brown rice.

VIRTUOUS VEGETABLE SOUP

This delicious, hearty soup is very versatile. You could get many meals out of it. You could remove some of the vegetables with a slotted spoon and serve them over brown rice or other cooked grains as a stew. You could add a shredded cooked chicken breast or a piece of firm fish like haddock. You could even use the vegetables in an omelet.

4 to 6 servings

2 tablespoons olive oil
½ small onion, peeled and sliced thin
1 celery stalk, sliced thin
1 large carrot, peeled and sliced thin
1 medium parsnip, peeled and sliced thin
2 garlic cloves, peeled and chopped
2 leeks (white and light green parts only), sliced thin and
     thoroughly rinsed to remove all grit
1 cup chopped kale
1 cup chopped collard greens
1 cup finely chopped cabbage
1½ cups diced canned no-salt tomatoes, with juice
2 cups cooked great northern beans (see page 258, or use
     organic beans in BPA-free cans), drained
1 quart unsalted vegetable broth or water
1 teaspoon dried thyme
1 bay leaf
Grated Parmesan or Romano cheese (optional)

1. Heat the oil in a large pot over medium-high heat. Add the onion, celery, carrots, parsnips, garlic, and leeks and cook until the carrots and parsnips are tender, stirring from time to time.

2. Stir in the kale, collards, and cabbage. Reduce the heat to low and cover the pot. Cook until the greens are wilted and soft.

3. Stir in the tomatoes, beans, broth, thyme, and bay leaf. Increase the heat and bring to a boil. Reduce the heat to medium-low and simmer for at least 30 minutes to allow the flavors to blend.

4. Remove the bay leaf. Serve immediately, sprinkled with a little cheese if you like. You can also turn off the heat and let the soup sit, covered, for an hour. Reheat over low heat before serving. Refrigerate any leftovers.

SPICY BEAN PARTY SOUP

This nutrition-packed soup will stick to your ribs. Start it in your slow cooker before you leave for work, and dinner will be waiting for you when you get home!

8 servings

3 cups chopped yams or sweet potatoes (no need to peel)
2 cups dried black beans
1 cup dried pinto beans
1 cup dried white beans
1 cup dried butter beans
1 cup chopped onion
2 teaspoons cayenne pepper
1 tablespoon no-salt vegetable seasoning
4 garlic cloves, peeled and finely chopped
¼ cup coconut water
2 quarts water
¼ cup chopped fresh parsley
¼ cup chopped fresh cilantro

1. Combine the yams, all the beans, the onion, cayenne, seasoning, and garlic in a large slow cooker. Pour in the coconut water and water, cover, and turn on low. Cook undisturbed for 8 hours, or until the beans are tender.

2. If the soup is too thick, add some boiling water to thin it. Stir the parsley and cilantro into the soup before serving. Refrigerate or freeze any leftovers.

GARLIC SOUP

4 servings

¼ cup coconut oil
8 garlic cloves, peeled and cut in half
¼ head cauliflower, cut up
1 teaspoon Bragg Liquid Aminos
½ teaspoon cayenne pepper
6 cups unsalted vegetable broth
1 lime, cut into 4 wedges

1. Heat the oil in a large pot over low heat. Add garlic cloves and cook, stirring from time to time, until the garlic is very soft. Do not let the garlic burn. If it starts to brown, remove the pot from the heat and let it cool down before returning to very low heat.

2. Add the cauliflower, liquid aminos, and cayenne, and stir to coat. Add the broth, increase the heat, and bring to a boil. Reduce the heat to low and simmer, stirring frequently, until the soup is soft and creamy.

3. Divide the soup among four bowls and drop a lime wedge into each bowl. Serve immediately.

CREAMY NUTMEG BROCCOLI SOUP

4 servings

1 quart unsalted vegetable broth
8 large broccoli stalks (florets and stems)
1 tablespoon coconut oil
½ cup scallions (green onions), chopped
1 or 2 garlic cloves, peeled and chopped
½ teaspoon ground nutmeg
⅛ teaspoon cayenne pepper
1 cup rice milk

1. Bring broth to a boil in a large pot over high heat. Add broccoli and reduce the heat. Cover and simmer until tender, about 10 minutes.

2. Meanwhile, heat the oil in a small skillet over medium heat. Add the scallions and garlic and cook until tender, stirring from time to time.

3. Stir the scallions and garlic into the broth. Remove from the heat and let cool for 10 to 15 minutes.

4. Working in batches, puree until smooth in a blender or food processor. Return the puree to the pot.

5. Combine the nutmeg and cayenne in a small bowl and stir in the rice milk. Gradually stir this mixture into the puree.

6. Return the soup to medium heat and cook until heated through, stirring from time to time. Serve hot.

CREAMY BUTTERNUT SQUASH SOUP

6 servings

3 tablespoons olive oil
2 onions, peeled and chopped
5 garlic cloves, peeled and chopped
1 quart unsalted vegetable broth
1 medium butternut squash, peeled, halved, seeded, and
   chopped
1 sweet potato, peeled and chopped
1 carrot, peeled and sliced thin
2 cups chopped white cabbage
2 packed cups baby spinach
⅓ cup very finely chopped fresh parsley
1 teaspoon cayenne pepper
Fresh thyme leaves, for garnish

1. Heat the oil in a large pot over low heat and cook the onions and garlic for 3 to 5 minutes, until soft but not colored.

2. Add the broth, squash, sweet potato, carrot, cabbage, and spinach. Bring to a boil, then reduce the heat and simmer for about 45 minutes, until the squash is soft.

3. Stir in the parsley and cayenne. Cover the pot and simmer for 15 minutes more.

4. With a slotted spoon, transfer about one-third of the vegetables to a blender or food processor. Puree until smooth. Stir the puree into the soup and reheat over low heat, stirring from time to time.

5. Sprinkle thyme leaves over each portion of soup just before serving.

Dinners

RED BEANS AND RICE CASSEROLE

Most cuisines have a version of beans and rice. The combination makes a complete protein.

4 servings

2 teaspoons olive oil
½ red onion, finely chopped
2 garlic cloves, peeled and very finely chopped
½ teaspoon Bragg Liquid Aminos
½ teaspoon cayenne pepper
1 teaspoon dried oregano
2 cups cooked red beans (see page 258, or use organic beans
    in BPA-free cans), drained
¼ teaspoon finely chopped seeded jalapeño chile
⅓ cup water
1 tablespoon tomato paste
⅓ cup pitted Spanish olives, chopped
2 tablespoons capers, rinsed
1 cup hot cooked long-grain brown rice

1. Heat the oil in a medium pot over medium heat. Add the onion and garlic and cook until the onion is translucent, stirring from time to time.

2. Stir in the liquid aminos, cayenne, oregano, beans, jalapeño, and 2 teaspoons of the water.

3. In a small cup, stir together the tomato paste and the remaining water. Stir into the beans, bring to a simmer, and cook for about 15 minutes to blend the flavors.

4. Stir in the olives and capers. Fold in the rice and serve immediately.

A Note on Cooking Beans

Beans are a very good source of protein. Since you will be limiting eating animal protein to three times a week, beans will become a staple of your diet. When you consider a recipe calling for beans, be aware that beans need to be soaked before cooking to reduce their gas-producing qualities, unless you cook them for hours in a slow cooker.

You can soak beans overnight if you plan in advance. The quickest way to soak and then cook beans is as follows:

1. Place beans in a sieve and rinse under cold running water. Remove any pebbles or debris.
2. Put the beans in a pot and cover with water by 2 inches. Bring to a boil over high heat and boil for 5 minutes.
3. Turn off the heat, cover, and let sit for 1 hour. The beans will soften and absorb water.
4. Drain the beans and rinse under cold running water. Return them to the pot and cover with 2 inches fresh water. Bring to a boil over high heat. Reduce the heat to medium and cook at a low boil until tender. Add more water to cover by 2 inches and bring back to a boil if the water boils too low. Test for doneness by taking out a bean with a slotted spoon and blowing on it; if the skin splits, taste it. You will feel when it is soft enough. This can take from 30 minutes to 2 hours or more, depending on the age of the beans.
5. Drain the beans, but save the broth for use in soups and other dishes. Store the beans in the refrigerator if not using right away, or freeze in a covered container.

If you find yourself short of time, you can use canned beans. Just make certain that the beans are organic and the can is BPA-free. Drain and rinse the beans before using. Cooking the beans yourself is preferred.

CITRUS SALMON WITH GREENS

This refreshing salad will become a favorite. You could substitute cooked shrimp for the salmon.

4 servings

½ cup Bragg Liquid Aminos
½ cup unflavored rice vinegar
3 tablespoons fresh orange juice
2 tablespoons flaxseed oil
1 teaspoon stevia
½ teaspoon cayenne pepper
3 garlic cloves, very finely chopped
2 skinless salmon fillets, about 10 ounces each
3 packed cups spinach, chopped
3 lemons, peeled, membranes removed, and flesh sectioned
1 large red onion, peeled and finely chopped

1. Preheat the oven to 350°F.

2. To make the dressing: Combine the liquid aminos, vinegar, orange juice, oil, stevia, cayenne, and garlic in a jar. Cover tightly and shake well until combined.

3. Place the salmon fillets in a baking dish. Brush very lightly with some of the dressing. Bake for about 20 minutes, until cooked through. Remove from the oven and let sit at room temperature to cool.

4. Place the spinach, lemons, and onion in a large bowl. Break the salmon into large flakes and add. Shake the remaining dressing well to recombine. Drizzle dressing over the salad and gently toss to coat. (You may not need all the dressing. Refrigerate any leftovers and use within 2 days.) Divide the salad onto four plates and serve.

TURKEY AMANDINE SALAD

This is a great recipe for leftover turkey, but you can start from scratch with turkey cutlets. The almonds add great crunch.

4 servings

1 teaspoon dried celery flakes
2 teaspoons no-salt vegetable seasoning
10 ounces organic turkey breast
½ cup nonfat plain Greek-style yogurt
2 teaspoons Bragg Liquid Aminos
1 teaspoon almond oil
½ cup chopped celery
½ cup finely chopped broccoli florets
¼ cup very finely chopped onion
1 packed cup organic spring lettuce mix
1 tablespoon raw organic almonds, chopped

1. Preheat the oven to 350°F.

2. Combine the celery flakes and seasoning and rub all over the turkey. Place the turkey in a small baking dish. Cover with foil and bake for 15 to 20 minutes. Remove from the oven, uncover, and set aside to cool to room temperature.

3. Stir together the yogurt, liquid aminos, and oil in a large bowl. Cut turkey into cubes. Add the turkey, celery, broccoli, and onion to the sauce and stir to coat. Cover and refrigerate for about an hour for the flavors to blend.

4. Add the lettuce and almonds and toss to combine. Serve immediately.

CURRIED CHICKEN SAUSAGE CASSEROLE

The aroma as this casserole cooks will make your mouth water.

4 servings

2 cups fully cooked organic chicken sausage (2 to 4 sausages),
   sliced ½-inch thick
2 cups chopped fresh tomatoes
1½ cups finely chopped kale
2 teaspoons curry powder
1 tablespoon no-salt vegetable seasoning
4 cups cooked lentils

1. Cook sausage in a large skillet over medium heat until lightly browned. Add the tomatoes, cover, and cook until the tomatoes are hot.

2. Meanwhile, steam the kale until soft. Drain when done.

3. Add the kale, curry powder, no-salt vegetable seasoning, and cooked lentils to the sausage and tomatoes. Cook until heated through.

LIME VEGGIE PASTA

This is an interesting twist on pasta that you are going to enjoy.

6 servings

2 teaspoons coconut oil
1 bunch scallions (green onions), trimmed and chopped
4 cups finely chopped white cabbage
3 cups sliced portobello mushrooms
1 cup sliced zucchini
8 ounces quinoa pasta
2 tablespoons very finely chopped garlic
2 tablespoons Bragg Liquid Aminos

4 teaspoons stevia
1 teaspoon cayenne pepper
4 large eggs, beaten
3 tablespoons fresh lime juice
1 teaspoon grated lime peel

1. Bring a large pot of water to a boil for the pasta.

2. Heat the coconut oil in a very large skillet over medium-high heat. Add the scallions, cabbage, mushrooms, and zucchini. Cook, stirring from time to time, until the vegetables are soft, about 10 minutes.

3. When the water comes to a boil, cook the pasta according to the package directions. Drain thoroughly in a colander.

4. Add the cooked pasta, garlic, liquid aminos, stevia, and cayenne to the vegetables. Cook, stirring from time to time, until everything is heated through.

5. Stir in the eggs and cook, stirring constantly, until the eggs are cooked through and completely coat the other ingredients.

6. Stir in the lime juice and peel and serve immediately.

ORANGE CHICKEN WITH SNOW PEAS AND ASPARAGUS

This recipe is so sophisticated you can serve it to company for an elegant meal.

4 servings

2 garlic cloves, peeled and very finely chopped
1 teaspoon grated orange peel
½ teaspoon dried thyme leaves, crushed
½ teaspoon dried rosemary leaves, crushed
⅛ teaspoon cayenne pepper

2 teaspoons no-salt vegetable seasoning
4 skin-on, bone-in chicken quarters (white or dark meat)
½ cup water
2 tablespoons cider vinegar
2 tablespoons Bragg Liquid Aminos
10 drops organic orange extract
2 tablespoons olive oil
1 bunch asparagus, trimmed
½ pound snow peas, trimmed

1. Heat a grill for indirect cooking, with the grate about 8 inches above the heat source.

2. Combine the garlic, orange peel, thyme, rosemary, cayenne, and 1 teaspoon of the seasoning in a small bowl. Slip your fingers between the skin and flesh of the chicken pieces, leaving the skin attached. Spread one-quarter of the spice mixture under the skin of each chicken piece. Pull the skin back over the spices.

3. In another small bowl, stir together the water, vinegar, liquid aminos, and extract to make a basting liquid.

4. Place the chicken on the prepared grill, skin side up. Cook for about 40 minutes, turning and basting the chicken every 5 minutes. The chicken is done when a fork can be inserted in the chicken with ease and the juices run clear.

5. When the chicken has been cooking for about 30 minutes, heat the oil in a large skillet over medium heat. Add the asparagus and snow peas. Cover and cook for about 5 minutes. Sprinkle with the remaining 1 teaspoon seasoning. Cover again and cook until the asparagus is tender, about 5 minutes more.

6. Serve the vegetables on the plate with the chicken.

SALMON WITH LEMON SAUCE AND VEGGIES

This dish is great to look at and even better to eat.

4 servings

1½ cups brussels sprouts (halved or quartered if very large)
1½ cups cauliflower florets
1½ cups chopped peeled carrots
4 skin-on 6-ounce salmon fillets
1 teaspoon no-salt vegetable seasoning
⅛ teaspoon cayenne pepper

For the lemon sauce
½ cup extra-virgin olive oil
2 tablespoons fresh lemon juice
2 tablespoons garlic powder
1 tablespoon dried oregano
2 teaspoons dried marjoram
½ teaspoon no-salt vegetable seasoning
½ teaspoon grated lemon peel
Pinch of cayenne pepper

1. Place the brussels sprouts, cauliflower, and carrots in a steamer basket over an inch or two of water in a large pot. Bring the water to a boil, cover the pot, and steam the vegetables until tender, about 10 minutes or less. Remove the vegetables from the steamer and set aside to keep warm.

2. Season the salmon with 1 teaspoon vegetable seasoning and ⅛ teaspoon cayenne pepper. Steam the salmon for 10 minutes or until it turns pink inside. Do not overcook! Remove the steamer basket from the pot and let excess moisture drain off the salmon.

3. While the salmon is cooking, make the lemon sauce. Combine the sauce ingredients in a small bowl and stir well to blend.

4. Divide the vegetables among four plates. Top each with a salmon fillet, and spoon lemon sauce over the top of the salmon. Serve immediately.

TURKEY CHILI OVER SPINACH FETTUCCINE

Turkey chili is always a hit. You might want to double the recipe and freeze the leftovers.

4 servings

1 tablespoon extra-virgin olive oil
1 yellow onion, peeled and finely chopped
2 garlic cloves, peeled and very finely chopped
½ pound ground turkey
1½ teaspoons chili powder
½ teaspoon dried oregano
¼ teaspoon cayenne pepper
Pinch of ground cumin
Pinch of ground cinnamon
1 cup unsalted vegetable broth
1 tablespoon tomato paste
1 teaspoon Bragg Liquid Aminos
1 cup cooked kidney beans (see page 258, or use organic
    beans in BPA-free cans), drained
1 small zucchini, finely chopped
1 carrot, peeled and grated
10 ounces uncooked spinach fettuccine
¼ cup chopped fresh cilantro

1. Bring a large pot of water to a boil for the pasta.

2. Heat the oil in a large skillet over medium heat. Add the onion and garlic and cook, for about 5 minutes, stirring from time to time. Add the turkey and cook until browned, stirring

to break up large clumps. Stir in the chili powder, oregano, cayenne, cumin, and cinnamon and cook for 2 or 3 minutes.

3. In a small bowl, stir together the broth, tomato paste, and liquid aminos. Stir into the chili. Stir in the kidney beans, zucchini, and carrot. Simmer for 15 minutes, stirring to make sure the mixture does not stick.

4. Cook the pasta according to the package directions. Drain in a colander.

5. Stir the cilantro into the chili. Divide the fettuccine among four bowls and top with the chili.

Dessert Smoothies and Desserts

If you have a sweet tooth, treat yourself to one of these. But be warned: you stand a good chance of gaining weight if you have a smoothie every day.

ORANGE CREAMSICLE SMOOTHIE

1 serving

¼ cup rice milk (preferably Rice Dream) or nondairy frozen
   yogurt
¼ cup crushed ice (if using rice milk)
1 scoop vanilla protein powder
½ teaspoon organic orange extract
¼ teaspoon organic vanilla extract

Combine all the ingredients in a blender and blend until smooth, 15 to 20 seconds.

CHOCOLATE BANANA SPLIT SMOOTHIE

1 serving

½ cup rice milk (preferably Rice Dream)
2 scoops chocolate protein powder
¼ cup crushed ice
½ teaspoon organic banana extract

Combine all the ingredients in a blender and blend until smooth, 15 to 20 seconds.

MOCHA SHAKER

1 serving

1 cup almond milk
¼ cup crushed ice
2 scoops chocolate protein powder
1 teaspoon stevia
¼ teaspoon organic coffee extract
¼ teaspoon organic vanilla extract

Combine all the ingredients in a blender and blend until smooth, 15 to 20 seconds.

PEPPERMINT FREEZE SMOOTHIE

1 serving

½ cup vanilla soy milk
¼ cup ice
½ cup nondairy vanilla frozen yogurt
1 scoop chocolate protein powder
⅛ teaspoon organic peppermint extract

Combine all the ingredients in a blender and blend until smooth, 15 to 20 seconds.

ALMOND CHOCOLATE SMOOTHIE

1 serving

1 cup almond milk
¼ cup crushed ice
1 or 2 scoops chocolate protein powder
1 teaspoon stevia
¼ teaspoon organic vanilla extract

Combine all the ingredients in a blender and blend until smooth, 15 to 20 seconds.

ANTIOXIDANT BERRY POPSICLES

These popsicles will satisfy your sweet tooth. Experiment with popsicles. They are a great snack.

6 to 8 servings

2 teaspoons organic unflavored gelatin powder
6 ounces boiling water
½ cup blueberries
½ cup strawberries

½ cup nonfat plain Greek-style yogurt
1 tablespoon stevia, or to taste
1 teaspoon organic vanilla extract

1. Combine the gelatin and water in a blender. Blend until the gelatin is completely dissolved.

2. Add the blueberries, strawberries, yogurt, stevia, and vanilla. Blend until thick, not runny.

3. Pour into Popsicle molds, add the sticks, and freeze for two hours

CINNAMON VANILLA APPLESAUCE

2 servings

1 tablespoon olive oil
2 cups chopped organic unpeeled apples
1 teaspoon stevia
⅛ teaspoon ground cinnamon
⅛ teaspoon ground nutmeg
⅛ teaspoon ground allspice
¼ cup water
⅛ teaspoon organic vanilla extract

1. Heat the oil in a skillet over medium heat. Add the apples and cook until lightly browned, stirring from time to time.

2. Stir together the stevia, cinnamon, nutmeg, and allspice. Sprinkle over the apples and stir to coat.

3. Add water a little at a time and cook until the apples are soft and the sauce is chunky. You may not need all the water. Add the vanilla when the sauce is done. Let cool a little to serve hot, or cool until just warm, or chill to serve cold.

DAD'S SOUTHERN RICE PUDDING

4 servings

2 cups almond milk
½ cup organic rice flour
2 tablespoons stevia
4 egg yolks, lightly beaten
2 cups cooked brown rice
2 teaspoons organic vanilla extract
¼ teaspoon Bragg Liquid Aminos
Slivered organic almonds, for garnish
1 teaspoon cinnamon

1. Combine the almond milk, flour, and stevia in a medium pot. Place over medium-low heat and cook, stirring constantly to prevent sticking, until the mixture comes to a boil. Reduce the heat and simmer for 2 to 3 minutes, stirring constantly. If it gets too thick to stir, mix in a little water.

2. Remove the pot from the heat and stir a little of the mixture into the egg yolks to temper them. Stir the tempered yolks back into the hot mixture. Return the pot to medium-low heat and simmer for 2 minutes more, stirring constantly.

3. Stir in the brown rice. Cook for 2 minutes more, stirring constantly so the pudding does not stick to the bottom of the pan.

4. Remove from the heat and stir in the vanilla extract and liquid aminos.

5. Enjoy warm, or chill before serving. Top with almonds and a sprinkle of cinnamon before serving.

You've Done
Yourself Proud

Congratulations! You have taken a big step toward getting to your ideal weight, alleviating nagging physical problems, supercharging your energy, and restoring your optimism and joy. Just buying *1 Pound a Day* because you want to change deserves acknowledgment. You have a vision of how you want to look and feel. You are thinking of doing something about it. That is a big step. When the desire is stronger than any resistance you might feel, you will have a blueprint for turning your life around.

In these pages, you have met many detoxers and heard their stories. So many of them received our previous book as a gift and read it, but then procrastinated. Some responded with an initial burst of enthusiasm that petered out when they considered the commitment involved. Others dismissed the program, tossing the book aside with the thought, *Are they crazy? There is no way I am not going to chew for twenty-one days! I could never get through it.* Intimidated, they put the book on a shelf or a nightstand where it stayed as a reminder. That is fine. The intent was there.

When things got bad enough, they turned to the book with new resolve. In story after story, you have read how easy it was for them to transform themselves once they had reached a tipping point. The determination to break out of their rut and to stop the downward spiral drove them to try.

Some of you may already be there. Your weight has risen steadily no matter what you do. Your health is deteriorating in little or big ways. You are tired and stressed. You do not want to resign yourself to never feeling well or to the image you see in photos or the mirror. Maybe you are beginning to get sick. You are ready to take control. If you follow the detox and transition, the changes you experience will surprise and delight you.

What is important to take away from this book is an understanding of how to eat for the rest of your life to ensure permanent weight loss and lasting health. Your body is a miraculous, complex creation. It demands so little of you. You owe your body protection from the toxins that are poisoning it on a cellular level. Dr. Roni's Healthy Eating Plan will guide you to nourish your body optimally. We have explained the principles behind the plan to give you even more motivation to eat right. Knowing why you are doing something can strengthen your commitment.

We are eager to hear from you about how your detox goes. There is a large community of detoxers who are generous with their tips and advice. You will find the "we are in this together" attitude very supportive. Check out our website (www.mvdietdetox.com) regularly for updates and links to our social media pages. We want to hear your stories and will answer your questions.

> Thank you very much! You've changed my body to the way it was before I had kids! It's amazing. Everyone who knows me couldn't believe that it was possible, but it is. And you have led me to this. You are the only one whose way worked for me. I'd tried everything before I bumped into your book. What you do is brilliant by guiding us through and following up consistently using Facebook. I've felt you're holding my hand through the detox days, which were not easy for me, but you made it bearable, and I felt joy and great support.
>
> N.M.

Our success is measured in the number of years our followers and fans have been with us. We strive to keep bringing you new information on the subject of detoxification. We listen to you. We will stay together on the cutting edge of detoxification and healthy lifestyle practices. We intend to keep educating you and listening to your concerns. Our goal is to help you work toward a healthier lifestyle by staying clean. We will continue to stay current and to share that knowledge with you. As we turned this manuscript in to our publisher, we were already considering several ideas for our next book. We will keep you posted on how our new project progresses. In the meantime, we wish you a smooth and transforming detox and a lifetime of healthy eating. *1 Pound a Day* will help you to lose weight, look great, lighten up, and stay that way.

ACKNOWLEDGMENTS

I would like to acknowledge my coauthor and business partner James Hester, a relentless hard worker who is passionately dedicated to getting our healing message out to the world. He has been a perfect client from the start, learning everything he could and never taking no for an answer. He stands for the truth, and I will always honor that.

Also, thanks to Diane Reverand, a brilliant writer and editor who has given so much to this project. She has taught me even more about support and team building in the short time I have known her.

To my private clients, retreaters, and friends from around the globe who have come to the Martha's Vineyard Holistic Retreat during the last sixteen years: THANK YOU! It has been an honor and a privilege to assist you on your journey to abundant health and healing. It has been a joy to answer your health questions, listen to your concerns, and facilitate your healing processes. I will continue to be committed to your health and vitality—it brings me such joy to see you thrive.

I would also like to thank my special retreat friends, who inspire me each and every day both professionally and personally. Thank you, Susan Swartz, Robin Quivers, Theophilus Nix Jr., Gail Rosenberg, Dr. Lorna Andrade, Dr. Enid Haller, and all the rest—you know who you are.

I also must acknowledge my retreat team, without whom this book would never be possible. To Dr. Linda Hicks PhD, ND,

Dr. Thomas Redner MD, Pamela Ray CCT, Linda Silva, Erin Bayer, Natalie Dickerson, Ariel Fixler, Virginia Campbell, and Dr. Makeba Moring PhD, ND—you are the best! You may all come from different walks of life, but you all have some things in common—huge hearts and a passion for healing. This is what the retreat runs on.

Thank you to the community of Martha's Vineyard for your support, especially Waterside Restaurant, for being my kitchen and meeting place; Blissed Out Juice Bar, for feeding us organic juices; Hollywood Spa, for bringing out the best in me; Peter and Ronni Simon, for jewelry; and Laughing Bear, for all my "last-minute outfits."

To my father, mother, and siblings, who all play a part in my daily life—thank you for keeping me strong. Family is connected heart to heart, and my mom, Lola Johnson, has created that special connection in all of us. Thank you to my sister, Jamie Johnson Harper, for always lending a helping hand at the retreat.

A message to my loving, smart, and tolerant kids, Toron DeLuz, Whitney Singh, and Tony DeLuz Jr.: You are the light that makes my day shine. And Tony Sr., you are the glue that keeps the family together.

I could not do all that I do without my Christian family prayers and Pastor Marcia Buckley. I give praise to God and thank Him daily for every breath that I take.

Dr. Roni DeLuz

*   *   *

First and foremost, I give all the praise and glory to God.

My partner, coauthor, my sixth woman and friend, Dr. Roni DeLuz, I came as a client in April 2003 and stayed till we hit the *New York Times* bestseller list. I heard God speak on the third day at your retreat back in 2003: "I will heal you, but pass my healing on to those in need." We obeyed. As loyal and diligent partners, we marched through every NO together. You are an angel. I always say, "Dr. Roni not only changed my life, but she saved it." I promised you the world would know about your life-changing work. We are doing it one person at a time. Everyone should have Dr. Roni in his or her home. Here's to getting the world healthy!

Pastor Marcia Buckley, my seventh woman . . . words cannot fit on this page to express the love and respect I have for you. You are a force, a God-loving and praying woman. You took me down in the water on day seven of my detox on Easter Sunday 2003, and my life has forever changed. I always refer to your church as "Little Church Big Miracles." If anyone is looking for a miracle, visit the Martha's Vineyard Apostolic House of Prayer.

Diane Reverand, I cannot thank our agent, David Vigliano, enough for bringing us together. I loved and respected you from the first day we met. You are a brilliant woman. Thanks for believing in our brand and sharing your insight on our book from day one. You never gave up. You are the best.

My family: Loretta, my mom; Jim, my dad; Judi and Michelle, the best sisters a brother could ask for; Aunt Joanie, Aunt Geri, Aunt Ann, Tommy Thompson, and all my family . . . thanks for all your encouraging love and support. R.I.P., Al Zelenka and Geff Walsh.

My extended family: Butch and Regina (my first woman) Woolfolk, Maye James (my second woman), Bethann Hardison (my fourth woman), Cathy Hughes (my fifth woman) Donna Fuimes, Lorainne Van Rensalier, Alvaro, Lino Pastrana, Father Chris, Judy

Myers, Judy Moskowitz, Sondra "Miss Everything" Fortunato, Sam Watkins, Lopez Brown, Cindi Gomes, Lisa Cortes, Marianne Trudel, Relinda Vasquez, Marvet Britto, John Meade, Rebecca Hunstman, Bishop Campbell, Gina Franano, Paris Gordon, Ted "Grandad" Doughty, Helena and Michael Doughty, Deborah Cooper, Barbara and Andrew Pace, Anel Pla, Tyrone Barrington, Linda Salvador and Al, Kathie "High Voltage" Dolgin, Tony Wyllie, Gene and Toni Burroughs, Arlene Weiss, Mareann Larsen, Patti Firincelli, the best detoxer in the world—you look great—Reno and Lynn Rolle, Timolin Cole.

And my dear sister Lucy Doughty and her beautiful husband, Nigel Doughty R.I.P. Thanks for inviting me into your family.

Our media family that believed in our detox and completed it: Steve Harvey, Robin Quivers, Tim Sabean, the Howard Stern family, Mikki Taylor, CBS news Cindi Gomes, Bill Fellings, Michelle Miller, Jamie Foster Brown, Flo Anthony, Loanne Parker, Annette Freeman, Pam El, Tracey Cloyd.

Our Simon & Schuster family: Jeremie Ruby-Strauss, what a pleasure, so smart; Jen Bergstrom, thanks for believing in us, we won't let you down; Jennifer Robinson, Kristin Dwyer, Heather Hunt, and the crew that completed *1 Pound a Day*. Thank you for your belief, support, leadership, and professional approach to our project. You are all such a star team.

Our agent, David Vigliano. Roni and I adore you; you are one of a kind, a legend. Anthony Mattero, you're a force on the rise; great things are in your very near future. Thanks for everything.

Jacqueline "Sergeant" Malloy, you are the best. Thanks for hanging in and keeping us together at corporate headquarters. Barbara Burns. Our wonderful attorney, Sol Slotnik; I know you love Diane . . . and you should, what a woman! Victoria Wilson, we adore you—thank you for all your help. The wonderful ladies at the Martha's Vineyard Holistic Retreat—Lindy, Pam and Linda—you are magical, healing women who care about people changing their lives.

My Martha's Vineyard crew: Amy Goldson, Kathy "Lola" and Paul, Gina and the Art Cliffs girls, Skip and Karen Finley, Marco Roean, Lisa Campbell, Dream Hampton, Suzanne de Passe, Susan and Jim Swartz, Jason Peringer (best massage therapist), Josh Montoya, (best Thai/yoga therapist), Besty Shands (best reflexologist), Mark McCan, Windmills Vitamin family, Keith Frankel, Jon Wiesgal, Angela Van Housten, Bev K, Ivette Tirin, Marva and Judy Mason . . . thank you all for everything you do with us . . . the best team ever!!!

Thank you, Doug Evans of Organic Ave, Marcus Antebi of Juice Press, James White of Jamba Juice, and Howard Schultz of Evolution, for bringing live, fresh juices into the bodies of millions; you are all angels. All the way to the top. The new drinks have arrived.

I dedicate this book to my six boys: Cole and Kyle Thompson, Jarrel and Troy Woolfolk, Sean and Lucas Doughty. I love you all very much. You are all growing into such fine men and little men. You all have great parents. Always follow their love and guidance. The lessons you learn in the valley are far more important than the ones on the peak.

Leon de Juda, thanks for inviting me into your sacred den; the five days were a magical and memorable experience I will treasure forever. Great things are destined for you.

Man's rejection is God's protection!

God Bless,
James Hester
Martha's Vineyard
⌒

INDEX

ABOUT THE AUTHORS

RONI DeLUZ founded the Martha's Vineyard Holistic Retreat in Vineyard Haven in 1997 to help others discover the optimal health she achieved after years of debilitating chronic illness. She is a registered nurse with a B.S. from Fairfield University. She has a PhD in natural health and a certificate as a naturopathic doctor from Clayton College of Natural Health/American Holistic College of Nutrition. She is a colonic hydrotherapist as well. She is recognized as a leading expert in the field of holistic health.

JAMES HESTER spent years working as a record company executive before a health crisis led him to Dr. Roni's retreat. She helped him lose more than forty pounds and turn his life around. He became so committed to her work that they became business partners and the authors of the *New York Times* bestseller *21 Pounds in 21 Days*.

Follow the authors on Twitter and Facebook by going to their website www.mvdietdetox.com.